Platelet-Vessel Wall Interactions in Hemostasis and Thrombosis

Synthesis Lectures on Integrated Systems Physiology— From Molecules to Function

Editor

D. Neil Granger, *Louisiana State University Health Sciences Center*
Joey P. Granger, *University of Mississippi Medical Center*

Physiology is a scientific discipline devoted to understanding the functions of the body. It addresses function at multiple levels, including molecular, cellular, organ, and system. An appreciation of the processes that occur at each level is necessary to understand function in health and the dysfunction associated with disease. Homeostasis and integration are fundamental principles of physiology that account for the relative constancy of organ processes and bodily function even in the face of substantial environmental changes. This constancy results from integrative, cooperative interactions of chemical and electrical signaling processes within and between cells, organs and systems. This eBook series on the broad field of physiology covers the major organ systems from an integrative perspective that addresses the molecular and cellular processes that contribute to homeostasis. Material on pathophysiology is also included throughout the eBooks. The state-of-the art treatises were produced by leading experts in the field of physiology. Each eBook includes stand-alone information and is intended to be of value to students, scientists, and clinicians in the biomedical sciences. Since physiological concepts are an ever-changing work-in-progress, each contributor will have the opportunity to make periodic updates of the covered material.

Platelet-Vessel Wall Interactions in Hemostasis and Thrombosis

Rolando E. Rumbaut and Perumal Thiagarajan

www.morganclaypool.com

ISBN: 9781615040391   paperback
ISBN: 9781615040407   ebook

DOI 10.4199/C00007ED1V01Y201002ISP004

A Publication in the Morgan & Claypool Publishers series
SYNTHESIS LECTURES ON INTEGRATED SYSTEMS PHYSIOLOGY—FROM MOLECULES TO FUNCTION

Lecture #4
Series Editor: D. Neil Granger, *Louisiana State University Health Sciences Center*
                      Joey P. Granger, *University of Mississippi Medical Center*
Series ISSN
Synthesis Lectures on Integrated Systems Physiology—
From Molecules to Function
Print 1947-945X   Electronic 1947-9468

Supported in part by grants from the Department of Veterans Affairs Research Service.

Platelet-Vessel Wall Interactions in Hemostasis and Thrombosis

Rolando E. Rumbaut and Perumal Thiagarajan
Michael E. DeBakey VA Medical Center and Baylor College of Medicine

*SYNTHESIS LECTURES ON INTEGRATED SYSTEMS PHYSIOLOGY—
FROM MOLECULES TO FUNCTION #4*

MORGAN & CLAYPOOL LIFE SCIENCES PUBLISHERS

ABSTRACT

Platelets are essential mediators of the physiologic process of hemostasis and pathologic thrombosis. While platelets do not interact with vascular walls under normal conditions, vascular injury or inflammation result in a coordinated series of events including platelet adhesion, aggregation, and promotion of coagulation. In this review, we describe the primary mechanisms involved in these responses in various vascular beds of both macro- and microvessels, and outline key unresolved aspects of these important interactions.

KEYWORDS

platelets, hemostasis, thrombosis, endothelium, microcirculation, microvesicles

Contents

CHAPTER 1

Introduction

Interactions of blood elements with vascular walls mediate the related processes of hemostasis and thrombosis. Hemostasis is the physiological arrest of hemorrhage at the site of vascular injury. It is orchestrated by the concerted response of platelets, the vessel wall and coagulation factors. Thrombosis refers to pathological formation of blood clots due to inappropriate activation of hemostatic mechanisms. Platelets are key blood components involved in these events; under physiologic conditions, platelets do not interact with blood vessels. However, in response to vascular damage, they promptly adhere to the damaged vessel wall at the site of injury, triggering a host of events that include recruitment of additional platelets (aggregation), leukocytes, and activation of blood coagulation [1]. While these events mediate cessation of bleeding and enable healing of wounds during "physiologic" hemostasis, these mechanisms also contribute to "pathologic" thrombosis that occurs in a variety of human illnesses, exemplified by atherosclerosis. Although hemostasis and thrombosis differ in their consequences, there is considerable overlap in the molecular mechanisms involved in these responses. We will review these mechanisms with an emphasis on platelets, and highlight intriguing differences between arterial and venous blood vessels, and between macro-and microvessels. The relevance of these processes to selected clinical entities will be outlined, as well as directions for future research in this important topic.

CHAPTER 2

General Characteristics of Platelets

2.1 OVERVIEW

Platelets were recognized as a distinct blood element in the late 19th century; the seminal work by Bizzozero in 1882 demonstrated that platelets (and not white blood cells) were responsible for formation of "white" clots at the sites of vascular injury in guinea pig microvessels *in vivo* [2]. As illustrated in those early descriptions, platelets are considerably smaller than the other previously recognized blood elements, erythrocytes and leukocytes. Mammalian platelets are anucleated cells arising from cytoplasmic fragmentation of megakaryocytes in the bone marrow, and have a typical diameter of ~2–3 μm. Platelets circulate in a discoid form (see Figure 2.1) and their average lifespan in humans is ~10 days [3]. However, following activation, they undergo dramatic changes in shape and ultrastructure; the membranes become ruffled with cytoplasmic projections and the granules are centralized and discharged [4,5]. Normal human platelet count is ~150,000–400,000/μl, though spontaneous bleeding resulting from reduced (but functionally normal) platelets is unusual at levels >10,000/μl [6].

Despite their lack of a nucleus, platelets are actively involved in a broad range of physiologic and pathologic processes. Platelets contain a variety of mediators that regulate hemostasis and thrombosis as well as a myriad of other functions including recruitment of other cells (chemotaxis), vasomotor function, cell growth, and inflammation, among others. Relevant constituents for thrombosis are present both on the cell membrane and in the cytoplasm, mainly within platelet granules. The platelet membrane, which consists of a typical bilayer of phospholipids, contains membrane glycoproteins that interact with various ligands, either soluble ligands that activate the platelets, or fixed ligands within the vessel wall or on other cells through which the platelets adhere to these structures. One unique feature of the platelet is that its plasma membrane contains a network of numerous invaginations into the platelet interior, connected to the exterior through small pores [7,8], known as the open canalicular system (OCS). This feature imparts upon the platelet a much greater surface area than would normally be found on such a small cell. Platelets contain a second channel system, derived from megakaryocyte smooth endoplasmic reticulum, known as the dense tubular system (DTS). The DTS stores calcium and a variety of enzymes involved in platelet activation; in contrast to the OCS, the DTS does not associate with the plasma membrane [9,10].

Platelet granules serve as secretory vesicles, releasing components to the extracellular fluid and also serve to direct molecules to the plasma membrane in a process of exocytosis. Three main pop-

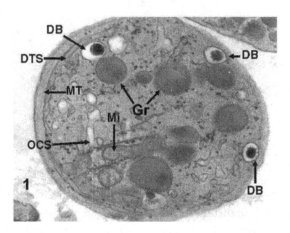

Figure 2.1: Transmission electron microscopy image of a resting human platelet, revealing many granules (Gr), several dense granules (DB, or dense bodies), the open canalicular system (OCS), and the dense tubular system (DTS). The image also depicts glycogen (Gly), some mitochondria (Mi) and a circumferential band of microtubules (MT). From reference [5], with permission.

ulations of granules are evident in unactivated, normal platelets, which differ in their ultrastructure, granule contents, kinetics of exocytosis, and function.

2.2   PLATELET GRANULES

2.2.1   ALPHA GRANULES

Alpha (α) granules are the largest ($\sim$200–400 nm) and most prevalent and heterogenous platelet granules [11]. There are about 50–60 granules per platelet, and they are responsible for the granular appearance of the cytoplasm in peripheral blood smears (stained with Romanowsky stains). These granules contain the majority of platelet factors involved in hemostasis and thrombosis. These include large polypeptides such as thrombospondin, P-selectin, platelet factor 4 and beta thromboglobulins as well as several factors involved in coagulation (Factors V, XI, XIII, fibrinogen, von Willebrand factor and high molecular weight kininogens). α-granules also contain a variety of adhesion molecules involved in platelet-vessel wall interaction such as fibronectin and vitronectin. The membrane of α-granules contains several proteins that are also expressed on the platelet cell membrane such as GPIb complex, GPVI, GP IIb/IIIa, and P-selectin. In addition, α-granules contain proteins involved in inflammation, wound healing, mitogenic growth factors (including platelet-derived growth factor, vascular endothelial growth factor, and transforming growth factor-β, among others) and a broad range of chemokines. Our understanding of platelet α-granule constituents is evolving; for example, a recent proteomic analysis of α-granules revealed the presence of 284 non-redundant proteins, of which 44 had not been described previously in these granules [12]. Further, α-granules demonstrate heterogeneity in their constituents and specific sub-populations of these granules may be released in response to various agonists [13, 14]. Understanding the mechanisms of differential release of α-granules, and the broad range of effects induced by release of their numerous constituents is an area of active investigation.

Secretion of α-granules during platelet activation is a complex process, involving coalescence in the platelet center, fusion of granules with the OCS and each other, as well as fusion with the plasma membrane [11, 15–17]. Platelets contain the complex machinery for granule release, including SNARE (soluble NSF [N-ethylmaleimide-sensitive factor] attachment protein receptors) and associated proteins and membrane lipids [17, 18]. Some α-granule constituents, such as P-selectin, exert their main physiologic role following their incorporation into the platelet membrane [19]. Other granule constituents exert their role following release from granules and participate in platelet aggregation, thrombosis, platelet adhesive interactions with leukocytes and other substrates, and regulation of cell proliferation via release of various growth factors. Deficiency of platelet α-granules occurs in a rare inherited disease, Gray Platelet syndrome (GPS), associated with quantitative and qualitative platelet dysfunction and a bleeding predisposition [20]. In GPS, proteins endogenously synthesized by megakaryocytes or endocytosed by platelets fail to enter α-granules of platelets due to abnormal formation of α-granules during megakaryocytic differentiation. This results in continued release of α-granule contents such as growth factors and cytokines into the bone marrow resulting in fibrosis (myelofibrosis). Morphologically, the platelets appear gray in peripheral smears.

2.2.2   DENSE GRANULES

Platelet dense granules are the smallest granules (~150 nm) and appear as dense bodies on electron microscopy (see Figure 2.1), due to their high calcium and phosphate content [9]. There are about 3–8 dense granules per platelet. In addition they contain high concentrations of adenine nucleotides and serotonin. Dense granules also contain small GTP-binding proteins and have been reported to contain relevant adhesion molecules present primarily on other platelet compartments including GPIb, GPIIb/IIIa, and P-selectin (discussed in separate sections). During platelet activation, dense granule membrane proteins incorporate with the platelet plasma membrane and granule contents are released into the extracellular environment. The released constituents contribute to recruit other platelets (aggregation) and also contribute to local vasoconstriction (e.g., serotonin). The ADP contained in dense granules is primarily involved in hemostasis and does not equilibrate with the metabolic pool of ADP, it is said to belong to the storage pool. Release of dense granules involves mechanisms comparable to those identified for α-granules, although the role of certain SNARE proteins have been reported to differ between the two granule populations [21]. The importance of dense granules to normal hemostasis is shown by the bleeding disorder in patients with deficiency of these granules. Platelet dense granule deficiency has been identified in two rare human conditions associated with predisposition to bleeding, Hermansky-Pudlak syndrome (HPS) and Chediak-Higashi syndrome [22]. HPS is defined by pigment dilution (affecting skin, hair, and eyes), resulting in oculocutaneous albinism, and platelet storage pool deficiency due to deficiency of dense granules. HPS is due to mutations in genes that mostly function in membrane and protein trafficking. There are eight known human HPS genes, each resulting in specific clinical variants of HPS [23]. Mouse strains that are deficient in orthologous genes also have been characterized and have a bleeding diathesis [24].

Chediak-Higashi syndrome is a rare autosomal recessive disorder characterized by oculocutaneous albinism, lymph node enlargement, hepatosplenomegaly (liver and spleen enlargement), and recurrent infections [22]. The CHS1/LYST gene on chromosome 1 affects the synthesis and maintenance of secretory granules within cells [25]. Lysosomes of fibroblasts, melanocytes, and hematopoietic cells, grossly enlarged to form giant lysosomes or vesicles [22]. In platelets, electron microscopy shows a large reduction in the number of dense granules but normal amounts of α-granules [26]. Platelet aggregation studies are consistent with deficiency in the storage pool of dense granule substances and suggest that this granule defect has an influence on the release mechanism of other granule constituents.

2.2.3   LYSOSOMES

Lysosomes represent the third category of platelet granules, with a size intermediate between α- and dense granules (~200–250 nm); they contain an intralumenal acidic pH with hydrolytic enzymes active towards a number of substrates including constituents of the extracellular matrix [9,27]. Due to similar electron density, lysosomes cannot be distinguished from α-granules in routine electron microscopy images such as those shown in Figure 2.1. However, they can be identified under electron microscopy with the use of cytochemical stains directed at enzymes contained in lysosomes such as acid phosphatase or arylsulfatase [28]. Platelet lysosome contents can be released upon activation, although their release requires greater stimulation than needed for release of α- and dense granules. Release of lysosomes involves mechanisms analogous to those involved in release of the other platelet granules [29,30]. While the functional role of platelet lysosomes is less well understood than that of α- and dense granules, lysosome release has been postulated to contribute to regulation of thrombus formation and remodeling of the extracellular matrix [9,27]. As in the case of α- and dense granules, lysosome release results in incorporation of lysosome proteins to the platelet plasma membrane; for example, platelet surface expression of lysosomal integral membrane protein (LIMP-1, or CD63) is used as a marker of significant (or "strong") platelet activation [31].

2.3   PLATELET ADHESION MOLECULES

Platelets contain a number of adhesion molecules both on the plasma membrane and within granules that are relevant for hemostasis and thrombosis, as well as cell-cell and cell-subendothelial matrix interactions (see Figure 2.2). The cellular localization and activation state of these molecules vary according to the state of platelet activation. The main adhesion molecules involved in hemostasis and thrombosis will be reviewed individually.

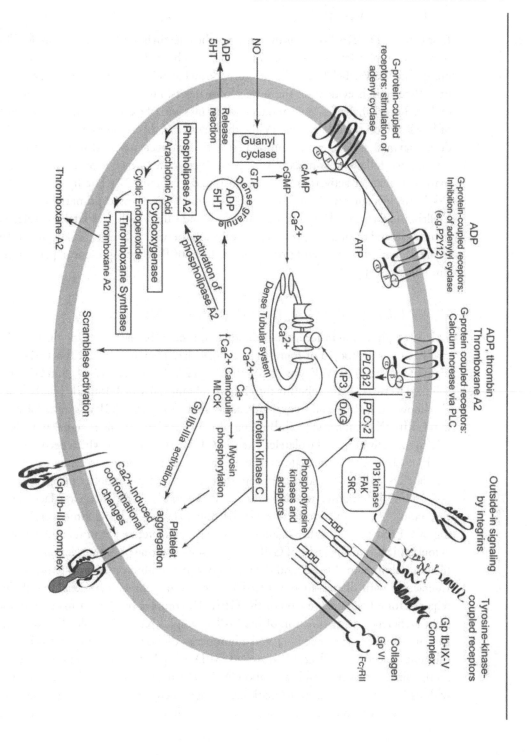

Figure 2.2: Schematic of the major platelet adhesion molecules and G-protein-coupled receptors and their signaling pathways; see text for details on individual molecules.

2.3.1   P-SELECTIN

P-selectin (CD62P, ~140 kd) is the largest of the selectin family of adhesion molecules. It is contained primarily on platelet α-granules, though has also been described on dense granules [32]; it is also present in the Weibel-Palade bodies of endothelial cells. Under resting, unstimulated conditions, little P-selectin is evident on the surface of platelets. However, following activation of platelets (or endothelial cells), the fusion of granule membranes with the cell membrane results in rapid expression of P-selectin on the cell surface. While the kinetics of this response varies according to agonist and dose, maximal surface expression of P-selectin has been reported to range from ~30 seconds to 10 minutes following stimulation [33, 34]. P-selectin surface expression is commonly used as a marker of platelet activation [19], as illustrated in Figure 2.3. The ligands for P-selectin include P-selectin glycoprotein ligand-1 (PSGL-1), which is expressed primarily on leukocytes [35], von Willebrand factor [36], glycoprotein Ibα [37] and sulfatides [38]. Platelet P-selectin contributes to hemostasis and thrombosis, as well as interactions between platelets, leukocytes and endothelial cells in inflammation [39]. In addition, a soluble form of P-selectin present in plasma may contribute to thrombosis [40].

2.3.2   GLYCOPROTEIN IB/IX/V (GPIB/IX/V)

This large glycoprotein receptor complex is the main platelet receptor for von Willebrand factor (vWF) and is composed of four distinct molecules. They include GPIbα (~145 kd), which is the main site for binding vWF, as well as GPIbβ (~22 kd), GPIX (~17 kd), and GPV (~82 kd). GPIbα is linked to two GPIbβ subunits through membrane-proximal disulfide bonds. The $\alpha/\beta 2$ complex, also known as GPIb, is non-covalently associated with GPIX (GPV is more loosely associated with two GPIb-IX complexes) [41]. Binding of vWF to GPIb initiates signal transduction events that lead to the activation of the platelet integrin GPIIb/IIIa ($\alpha_{IIb}\beta_3$), which becomes competent to bind vWF or fibrinogen to mediate platelet aggregation. In addition to being the main vWF receptor on platelets, GPIbα has also been reported to bind a large number of ligands, including thrombospondin [42], counter-receptors such as P-selectin [37], the integrin Mac-1 on leukocytes [43], thrombin [44], coagulation factors XII, XI, and VIIa [45–47], and kininogen [48]. However, binding of GPIbα to these other ligands is less well characterized than its interaction with vWF. The cytoplasmic C-terminal tails of GPIb contain several serine phosphorylation sites and interacts with filamin, calmodulin, 14-3-3, and the regulatory p85 subunit of the phosphoinositide 3-kinase [41]. Interaction with filamin links GPIb-IX-V to the membrane cytoskeleton; all three subunits are required for efficient expression of the GPIb-IX complex on the plasma membrane of transfected cells. Deficiency or dysfunction of the GPIb complex results in a bleeding disorder known as the Bernard–Soulier Syndrome [49], and a number of disease-causing mutations have been mapped to the genes encoding GPIbα, GPIbβ, and GPIX [50]. While this receptor is present constitutively on the platelet plasma membrane, and vWF is normally present in plasma, binding of the receptor with its ligand involves a conformational change in either or both components. These changes are induced by alterations in blood flow and the resultant shear stress, a concept discussed in greater

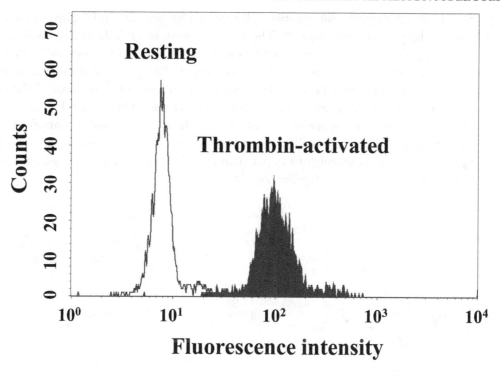

Figure 2.3: Flow cytometry of P-selectin expression on mouse platelets. Resting platelets reveal limited expression of P-selectin, whereas platelets incubated with thrombin (1 U/ml for 10 minutes) demonstrate significant P-selectin expression.

detail in Chapter 3. The antibiotic ristocetin induces these changes in the absence of shear stress and is used to assess this interaction *in vitro* [51].

2.3.3 GLYCOPROTEIN IIB/IIIA (GP IIB/IIIA)

Platelet GP IIb/IIIa ($\alpha_{IIb}\beta_3$) plays an essential role in platelet aggregation, and thus it has been studied most intensively. Like other integrins, it is a heterodimer with an alpha (α_{IIb}, ~136 kd) and a beta (β_3, ~92 kd) subunit. There are approximately 80,000 copies of GP IIb/IIIa on the surface of unstimulated human platelets, and additional molecules in the membranes of platelet granules are translocated to the platelet surface during platelet secretion [52]. This molecule is expressed constitutively on the plasma membrane as an inactive form in resting platelets, though undergoes conformational changes during activation. As depicted in Figure 2.4, this integrin is composed of a large extracellular nodular head with its ligand-binding site and flexible stalks containing its transmembrane (TM) and cytoplasmic domains [53,54]. The nodular head of the alpha subunit is folded into a β-propeller configuration, followed by a "thigh" and 2 "calf" domains, constituting the extracellular portion of the α_{IIb} stalk. The β_3 head consists of a βA-domain containing a metal ion-dependent adhesion site (MIDAS) motif, as well as a hybrid domain whose fold is similar to that of I-set Immunoglobulin domains. The β_3 stalk consists of a PSI (plexin, semaphorin, integrin) domain, 4 tandem epidermal growth factor (EGF) repeats, and a unique carboxyterminal βTD domain. In the resting stage, the head region is severely bent over in a compact "V" shape (Figure 2.4). Activation induces a change in the shape of the headpiece, shifting the α_{IIb} and β_3 domains from a closed conformation with adjacent stalks to an open conformation with stalks separated, exposing the ligand binding site, consisting of a β_3 βA-domain and forming a "cap" composed of 4 loops on the upper surface of the α_{IIb} β-propeller domain.

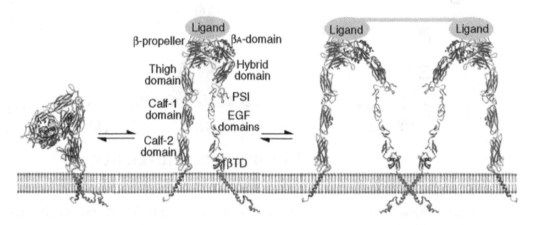

Figure 2.4: Model of platelet integrin $\alpha_{IIb}\beta_3$ (GPIIb/IIIa), and conformational changes induced following activation. The inactive "V"-shaped compact form is shown on the left. Binding of a ligand results in extension of the molecule into its active state (middle panel), and subsequent clustering of GPIIb/IIIa molecules (right panel). According to the model, these states exist in equilibrium. From reference [53], with permission.

Platelet GPIIb/IIIa can bind to fibrinogen, as well as other ligands such as vWF, fibronectin and vitronectin [55]. The key role of GP IIb/IIIa in platelet aggregation is discussed in Chapter 4; this molecule represents a major target for directed therapy in patients with thrombotic disorders [56].

2.3.4 COLLAGEN RECEPTORS

As reviewed in Chapter 3, platelet interaction with subendothelial collagen is an essential step in primary hemostasis. The $\alpha_2\beta_1$ integrin and glycoprotein VI (GP VI, ~65 kd) are the primary collagen receptors; both play a prominent role in hemostasis. These receptors bind to specific sequences on collagen with different affinities [57]. $\alpha_2\beta_1$ binds to various sequences containing the GER (glycine-glutamic acid-arginine) triplet, while GPVI binds to sequences containing at least two

GPO (glycine-proline-hydroxyproline) triplets [58, 59]. Platelet adhesion promoted by integrin $\alpha_2\beta_1$ induces activation of platelet GPIIb/IIIa through the phospholipase C (PLC)-dependent stimulation of the small GTPase Rap1b [60]. Platelet GPVI is expressed constitutively on the platelet plasma membrane, and is also expressed on α-granules [61]. Following platelet activation, surface expression of GPVI increases and intracellular expression decreases, consistent with their release from α-granules and incorporation into the plasma membrane. GPVI belongs to the immunoglobulin superfamily that contains two C2 immunoglobulin-like domains and an arginine residue in the transmembrane region that forms a salt bridge with the aspartic acid residue of the Fc receptor γ (FcRγ)-chain [62]. Activation by collagen leads to phosphorylation of its immunoreceptor tyrosine-based activation motif (ITAM), leading to a sequence of events involving several adaptor proteins, and resulting in phosphorylation and activation of PLCγ2 [63,64]. GPVI mainly binds to collagen types that can form large collagen fibrils such as collagen type III. GPVI is a key adhesion molecule involved in hemostasis and thrombosis; absence of GPVI in humans is associated with a predisposition to bleeding [65].

2.4   G-PROTEIN-COUPLED RECEPTORS

2.4.1   THROMBIN

Thrombin is a key component of the blood coagulation cascade and a potent stimulator of platelets. Platelet responses to thrombin are mediated by protease-activated-receptors (PAR). PAR are unique among G protein-coupled receptors in that activation occurs through proteolytic cleavage of the receptor by thrombin and unmasking a specific ligand [66]. Thrombin binds to the extracellular domain of PAR-1 and PAR-4, which are then cleaved to form a new amino terminus with its tethered ligand; the tethered ligand activates the receptor and induces signaling. Synthetic peptides, called thrombin-receptor agonist peptides (TRAPs), mimic the new amino terminus and potently activate the thrombin receptor resulting in platelet activation, secretion, and aggregation independently of receptor cleavage. Both PAR-1 and -4 activation must be inhibited to prevent platelet activation subsequent to thrombin binding to platelets. In mouse platelets, PAR-3 and PAR-4 (as opposed to PAR-1 and PAR-4), mediate the response to thrombin [67, 68]. Human platelets also express PAR3, though in contrast to mice, PAR3 does not appear to contribute to platelet responses to thrombin [67, 69]. Thrombin signaling via either PAR1 or PAR4 induces platelet activation, shape change, and granule release; PAR1-dependent responses are evident at lower thrombin concentrations than those induced by PAR4 [67]. The signaling pathways downstream of PAR-1 and PAR-4 in human platelets are not entirely clear, though both PAR-1 and PAR-4 couple to G_q and $G_{12/13}$ G-proteins, resulting in activation of phospholipase C, calcium mobilization, and protein kinase C activation [70]. Thrombin receptor antagonists may represent a novel target for clinical antithrombotic therapy are undergoing large scale clinical trials [71].

2.4.2   ADENOSINE DIPHOSPHATE (ADP) AND ADENOSINE TRIPHOSPHATE (ATP)

ADP has long been recognized as a stimulus for platelet adhesion and aggregation, though with distinct features than the response to thrombin. Exposure of human platelets to low concentrations of ADP results in an initial reversible aggregation without granule release. Higher concentrations of ADP, induce release of granules and synthesis of prostaglandins giving rise to a characteristic biphasic response with irreversible aggregation.

The response to ADP on human platelets is mediated by G-protein coupled P2Y receptor family of G protein-coupled, seven transmembrane domain receptors (P2Y1 and P2Y12). The P2Y1 receptor couples to G_q and mobilizes intracellular calcium ions to mediate platelet shape change and aggregation. The P2Y12 receptor is coupled to the inhibition of adenylyl cyclase through G_i and it is the target of antithrombotic agents, such as ticlopidine, clopidogrel, and prasugrel [72]. Mutations in the P2Y12 receptor are associated with a life-long bleeding disorder [73]. ATP is a less potent stimulus than ADP, but results in platelet activation, shape change, and enhances platelet responses to other agonists such as collagen; ATP-induced signaling occurs via a ligand-gated ion channel (P2X1) [74].

2.4.3   PROSTANOIDS

Thromboxane A_2 (TXA_2) is a product of arachidonic acid metabolism; two isoforms of thromboxane receptors have been described: $TP\alpha$ and $TP\beta$, though the $TP\alpha$ is the predominant isoform expressed on human platelets [74,75]. TP is also a member of the G protein-coupled receptor (GPCR) family and is shown to be coupled with G_q and G_{13}, resulting in phospholipase C activation and RhoGEF activation, respectively [76]. TXA_2 is released by various cells, including platelets, where it acts in an autocrine and paracrine manner. TXA_2 results in platelet shape change, aggregation, degranulation and enhancement of response to other agonists, thus amplifying platelet activation. Inhibition of TXA_2 production (by inhibition of cyclooxygenase-1) is one of the mechanisms of action of aspirin, a commonly used antiplatelet agent [56, 77, 78], and direct inhibitors of TP-α are undergoing evaluation for potential clinical use [79]. Platelets express receptors for other prostanoids, including prostacyclin (which mediates inhibition of platelet aggregation) and prostaglandin E_2 (which has a biphasic effect on platelets).

CHAPTER 3

Platelet Adhesion to Vascular Walls

3.1 ADHESION TO SUBENDOTHELIUM FOLLOWING VASCULAR INJURY

Under physiologic conditions, platelets circulate preferentially in close proximity to vascular walls [80, 81]. However, they do not interact with endothelial cells, which provide a natural resistance to thrombosis. When the continuity of endothelial layer is disrupted and the underlying subendothelial matrix is exposed, a coordinated series of events are set in motion to seal the defect, as depicted in Figure 3.1. Platelets play the primary role in this process, and various substrates may mediate their adhesion to the vascular wall in response to injury.

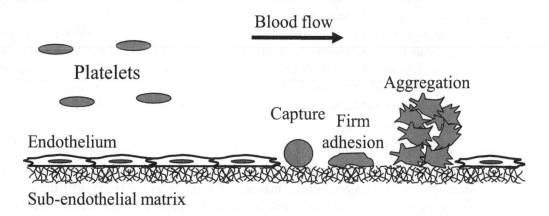

Figure 3.1: Cartoon illustrating the sequence of events involved in platelet-vessel wall interactions following vascular injury. Resting platelets circulating in discoid shape are shown on the left; vascular injury (depicted as endothelial denudation) results in capture of platelets, firm adhesion to the subendothelium and platelet shape change. Recruitment of additional platelets (platelet-to-platelet adhesion, or aggregation) is depicted on the right. See text for details.

3.1.1   VON WILLEBRAND FACTOR (VWF)

A key initial step in platelet adhesion to the site of injury involves interactions between the GP Ib-IX-V complex and the A1 domain of vWF in the exposed subendothelium [1,82,83]. vWF is a multimeric protein synthesized by endothelial cells and megakaryocytes; it is contained in Weibel-Palade bodies of endothelial cells, α-granules of platelets, in soluble form in plasma, as well as in the subendothelial matrix [84]. Immobilized vWF is sufficient to initiate platelet adhesion under flow, though the kinetics of these interactions vary according the hydrodynamic conditions [85]. A main determinant of the role of vWF on platelet adhesion is shear rate [85], which is a measure of the gradient of flow velocity relative to the distance from the vascular wall. Shear rate is a direct function of blood flow velocity and an inverse function of cross-sectional area, and is expressed in units of inverse seconds (s^{-1}). *Ex vivo* studies with human blood demonstrate that GPIb-vWF is the primary adhesive interaction initiating platelet adhesion at high shear rates (> 1000 s^{-1} [85]), as occur in arterial microvessels, or arterioles [86]. Analogous studies in mice (an increasingly studied experimental model of thrombosis) reveal comparable shear rate-dependence of GPIb-vWF-mediated adhesion occurring at higher shear rates [87]. Of note, in the presence of a significant reduction in vascular cross-sectional area (as may result from thrombus, atherosclerotic plaque, vasoconstriction, etc.), wall shear rates may increase substantially and GPIb-vWF interactions may predominate [88,89]. Shear rate is a determinant of shear stress, a force per unit area applied parallel to the vascular wall (frequently described in units of dyn/cm^2). The relevance of shear stress to platelet-endothelial interactions is discussed in Section 3.2.

In addition to its role in mediating platelet-vessel wall interactions, vWF also serves as the carrier molecule for coagulation factor VIII. The relevance of vWF in hemostasis and thrombosis is illustrated in humans by von Willebrand disease, a group of bleeding disorders characterized by varying degrees of vWF deficiency [90]. Similarly, mice with genetically induced vWF deficiency demonstrate delayed platelet interactions with vascular walls following injury [91,92].

3.1.2   COLLAGEN

Endothelial cells provide a barrier to the interaction of platelets in flowing blood with various types of collagen present in the subendothelial matrix [93]. The platelet receptors GPVI and $\alpha_2\beta_1$ mediate the interaction with collagen, though these interactions require platelet capture mediated by GPIb-vWF interactions. Both GPVI and $\alpha_2\beta_1$ mediate collagen-induced platelet activation under flow conditions, though the precise sequence of these interactions is not entirely clear. For example, some studies on human platelets *ex vivo* suggest that initial binding of GPIb complex to vWF results in a conformational change of the α subunit of collagen receptor $\alpha_2\beta_1$, enhancing its affinity to collagen [94], and subsequently enabling GPVI-collagen interaction. Others suggest an essential, cooperative role for both GPVI and $\alpha_2\beta_1$ in mediating platelet adhesion at the site of injury, with GPVI signaling first and subsequently activating $\alpha_2\beta_1$ [95]. Further, studies in mice with genetic deficiency of $\alpha_2\beta_1$ reveal discordant results, with reports of prolonged [95] as well as normal [96] bleeding response following transection of the tail (tail bleeding time). The relative contributions of

GPVI and $\alpha_2\beta_1$ to platelet interactions with collagen, and how they relate to GPIb-vWF mediated adhesion *in vivo* remain to be elucidated fully.

3.1.3   OTHER SUBENDOTHELIAL COMPONENTS

The subendothelium contains various other substrates capable of binding to and activating platelets, including laminin, thrombospondin, fibronectin, and vitronectin, among others [54,97]. These substrates may bind to the integrins described earlier ($\alpha_{IIb}\beta_3$ and $\alpha_2\beta_1$) as well as other β_1 and β_3 integrins. The relative role of each of these subendothelial matrix components in hemostasis and thrombosis is incompletely understood.

3.2   ENDOGENOUS MECHANISMS PREVENTING PLATELET ADHESION TO ENDOTHELIUM

The integrity of the endothelial lining provides a barrier preventing platelet adhesion to subendothelial substrates, and focal removal of endothelium (denudation) has long been studied as a mechanism of platelet adhesion to vascular walls. However, increasing evidence both *in vitro* and *in vivo* demonstrates that in response to various stimuli, platelets may adhere to the vascular endothelium in the absence of endothelial denudation. Various mechanisms prevent adhesion of platelets to endothelial cells under normal conditions; these are outlined below.

3.2.1   NITRIC OXIDE

Nitric oxide (NO) was initially discovered as an endothelial-derived relaxing factor [98,99]; it is now recognized to mediate a plethora of physiologic processes throughout a broad range of cells. NO is derived from L-arginine and oxygen in the presence of several cofactors; endothelial NO synthase (eNOS) is one of the three isoforms of NOS [100]. eNOS is expressed constitutively on endothelial cells though is activity may be regulated actively by a variety of mechanisms [101]. Endothelial cells may release NO in response to agonists binding to endothelial receptors (e.g., bradykinin, histamine, ATP, etc.) or by blood flow-induced shear stress. Many of the biological actions of NO released by endothelial cells, including vasodilatation, are mediated by activation of soluble guanylate cyclase resulting in increased intracellular cyclic guanosine monophosphate (GMP) [102]. NO has also been shown to exert physiologic roles via cyclic GMP-independent mechanisms, including nitrosylation of a host of target proteins [103]. The role of NO as an inhibitor of platelet adhesion and activation has been described in a number of models [100,104–107], although the mechanisms involved remain to be fully clarified. Both cyclic GMP-dependent and –independent mechanisms have been reported to contribute to the NO-induced inhibition of platelet adhesion and activation [105,108]. Although the antiplatelet actions of NO are well documented from experiments on isolated platelets, the relative contribution of endogenous NO as an inhibitor of platelet adhesion *in vivo* is not straightforward. Experimental models have examined this question using a variety of approaches, including inhibitors of NOS, pharmacologic agents that release NO, and mice with genetic deficiency of eNOS under various conditions, with evidence of discordant findings [107,109–111]. The role of NO on platelet adhesion *in vivo*, particularly under conditions associated with endothelial dysfunction, are likely highly complex. For example, the balance between NO and reactive oxygen species has been suggested as a key determinant of platelet adhesion in some experimental models [112]. Further, NO may also inhibit leukocyte adhesion to vascular endothelium [113], and this may impact leukocyte-dependent platelet adhesion to endothelium, as outlined in Section 3.3. Understanding the role of NO in platelet-endothelial adhesion *in vivo* is complicated further by conflicting reports on whether platelets express a functional form of eNOS [114–116].

3.2.2   PROSTACYCLIN

Prostacyclin (PGI_2) is the main product of arachidonic acid metabolism on endothelial cells, and shares some functional similarities with nitric oxide [117]. PGI_2 is also an endothelial-derived relaxing factor and is synthesized in response to various stimuli that release NO, including shear stress. Endothelial prostacyclin synthesis depends on cyclooxygenase-1 (COX-1) and prostacyclin synthase [118]. In addition to being a vasodilator, PGI_2 has long been known to be a potent inhibitor of platelet aggregation [119,120]. While the role of PGI_2 as inhibitor of aggregation is well established, fewer reports suggest an inhibitory effect on platelet adhesion on injured endothelium *in vivo* or in *ex vivo* experiments [121–123]. While NO signaling involves cyclic GMP, prostacyclin signaling involves cyclic adenosine monophosphate (AMP); NO and prostacyclin seem to have synergistic effects as inhibitors of platelet activation [118]. The effects of prostacyclin on platelets and blood vessels contrasts with that of another cyclooxygenase metabolite, thromboxane A_2, a vasoconstrictor and stimulator of platelet activation. A balance between these metabolites is presumed to be relevant for platelet activation *in vivo* and to mediate the beneficial effects of low-dose aspirin used clinically as an antithrombotic [118].

3.2.3   ECTO-ADENOSINE DIPHOSPHATASE (ADPASE)

Endothelial ecto-ADPase (CD39/nucleoside triphosphate diphosphohydrolase) is an integral component of the endothelial cell surface membrane; its antiplatelet effects are mediated by metabolizing ADP, which is a potent stimulator of platelet aggregation [124]. CD39 seems to inhibit platelet activation indirectly, and not via a direct interaction with platelets; this characteristic differs from the roles of NO and PGI_2 outlined above. A soluble form of CD39 has been demonstrated to exert antithrombotic effects in experimental models and has been proposed as a novel therapeutic approach in patients with thrombotic disorders [125].

3.2.4   ENDOTHELIAL SURFACE LAYER

The interface between flowing blood and endothelial cell membrane contains a hydrodynamically significant layer, composed mainly of glycoproteins and proteoglycans. This layer, known as glycocalyx, is increasingly recognized as a physiologically relevant structure in regulation of endothelial permeability, responses to shear stress, and leukocyte-endothelial interactions [126]. In addition, the glycocalyx may represent another endothelial mechanism preventing platelet adhesion, given its physical location, and experimental evidence of platelet adhesion to endothelium following disruption of the glycocalyx [127,128]. Precise determinations of glycocalyx dimensions in the vasculature are limited by the physical characteristics of the layer, which may be subject to alteration during processing for ultrastructural studies [129], such as those depicted in Figure 3.2. These characteristics likely result in the broad range of reported values, ranging from approximately 20 nm to nearly 1 μm [130–132]. The endothelial glycocalyx is currently an area of active investigation in endothelial biology and may become a target for therapeutic manipulations, including for its potential effects on platelet adhesion [127,133].

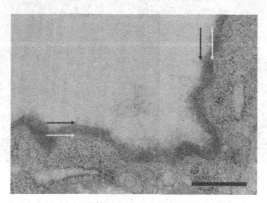

Figure 3.2: Transmission electron microscopy image of rat mesenteric microvascular endothelium, following perfusion with Alcian Blue, using techniques based on those described by van den Berg, et al. [129]. An electron dense layer is evident adjacent to the endothelial cell plasma membrane (white arrows) protruding into the vascular lumen (black arrows), with variable thickness, on average ~100 nm. Bar = 500 nm. Electron microscopy performed by Alan Burns, Ph.D., University of Houston, TX.

3.3   MECHANISMS OF PLATELET ADHESION TO ENDOTHELIUM

A variety of inflammatory states may result in platelet adhesion to endothelial cells in the absence of denudation, and without evidence of significant alterations in the endothelial integrity. These processes may result from inhibition of the endogenous mechanisms preventing platelet adhesion and/or by inducing endothelial release of molecules that promote platelet adhesion. Further, several of these inflammatory conditions result in leukocyte adhesion to endothelial cells, primarily in the post-capillary venules of the microcirculation, with presence of leukocyte-platelet adhesion at those sites.

Platelet adhesion to endothelial cells has been documented experimentally in a number of inflammatory states, including ischemia/reperfusion injury, exposure to endotoxin, sickle cell disease, and hypercholesterolemia, among others [39]. These studies frequently involve the technique of intravital video microscopy, by monitoring trafficking of exogenously administered fluorescent-labeled platelets in the microcirculation [134], as shown in Figure 3.3. Several mechanisms for platelet adhesion to endothelial cells have been suggested.

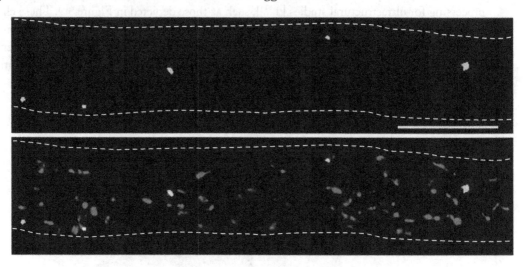

Figure 3.3: Adhesion of fluorescently-labeled platelets to endothelial cells of a mouse cremaster venule, under endotoxin-induced inflammation. Exogenous platelets were labeled with a fluorescein-based dye (green) and infused into a recipient mouse for monitoring *in vivo* during intravital microscopy (upper panel); dashed lines outlined the microvascular walls. Lower panel depicts red fluorescent staining of platelets in excised tissues, demonstrating endogenous (red) and exogenous (red+green, appearing yellow) labeled platelets. Approximately 8% of the total adherent platelets are exogenous, comparable to the percentage in peripheral blood (10%). Bar = 40 μm. Figure reproduced from reference [134], with permission.

3.3.1   ENDOTHELIAL P-SELECTIN-DEPENDENT MECHANISMS

Many of the inflammatory conditions noted above are associated with endothelial activation and release of P-selectin stored in granules known as Weibel-Palade bodies. Exposure of P-selectin on the surface of endothelium may promote platelet adhesion by binding to GPIb complex on platelets. This mechanism appears to mediate platelet adhesion in experimental models of sickle cell disease and endotoxemia [135,136].

Endothelial cell P-selectin also mediates the initial transient interactions of leukocytes with endothelial cells (rolling), which precedes their firm adhesion to endothelium. A counter-ligand on leukocytes is P-selectin glycoprotein ligand-1 (PSGL-1). In some inflammatory states, platelet adhesion to endothelium depends largely on leukocyte adhesion, since depletion of circulating neutrophils prevents adhesion of platelets. Leukocyte-dependent platelet adhesion has been documented in various models including ischemia/reperfusion injury, endotoxemia, hypercholesterolemia, and corneal wound injury [39, 137–139]. In many of these models, recruitment of leukocytes and platelets to vascular walls reveal marked temporal and spatial correlation, as shown in Figure 3.4. The adhesive mechanisms mediating platelet-leukocyte interactions in the various inflammatory states remain to be characterized fully. Platelet P-selectin-Leukocyte PSGL-1 is a likely mediator of platelet-leukocyte adhesive interactions [140]. However, several other mechanisms mediating these interactions have been proposed, including platelet GPIbα-leukocyte CD11b/CD18, platelet intercellular adhesion molecule-2 (ICAM-2)-leukocyte lymphocyte function-associated antigen-1 (LFA-1), and platelet junctional adhesion molecule-3 (JAM-3) and leukocyte macrophage antigen-1 (Mac-1) [43,140,141]. The relative contribution of the multiple potential mediators of platelet-leukocyte adhesive interactions in inflammatory disorders is unclear. Of interest, while leukocytes promote platelet adhesion in these models, evidence of platelets promoting leukocyte adhesion has been demonstrated experimentally, since depletion of circulating platelets markedly reduces leukocyte recruitment in various models [139, 142]. These findings suggest an elaborate inter-dependence between platelet and leukocyte adhesion to endothelium in inflammation, and represents an area of active investigation.

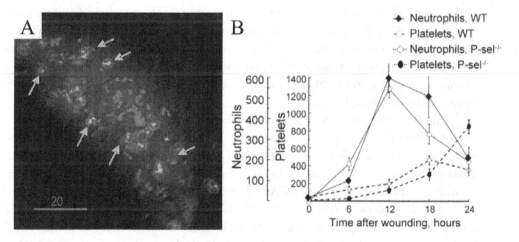

Figure 3.4: Platelet and leukocyte adhesion to endothelial cells *in vivo* in a mouse model of inflammation induced by corneal injury. A) Immunofluorescence of a venule in the corneal limbus, with abundant neutrophils (green) and platelets (red); the arrows depict examples of spatial correlation between platelets and neutrophils. Bar = 20 μm. B) Tight temporal correlation between platelet and neutrophil recruitment in the same model, in wild-type- (WT) and P-selectin-deficient mice (P-sel-/-). Panel A figure courtesy of C. Wayne Smith (Baylor College of Medicine, Houston, TX), panel B figure reproduced from reference [139], with permission ©The Association for Research in Vision and Opthalmology.

3.3.2   ENDOTHELIAL VWF-DEPENDENT MECHANISMS

Endothelial vWF is also stored in Weibel-Palade bodies, and is released in response to similar stimuli as those that induce endothelial P-selectin release. The newly released form of vWF is larger and more adhesive than vWF present in plasma, also known as ultralarge (UL) vWF. This multimeric form is normally cleaved by the plasma metalloprotease, ADAMTS-13 [143]. The ULVWF anchors to the endothelial surface in part by P-selectin, and promotes platelet adhesion via interaction with GPIb complex on platelets [36,143,144]. In the absence of cleavage, the ULVWF multimers result in long string-like structures, which support platelet adhesion with a "beads-on-a-string" appearance [145]. Figure 3.5 illustrates platelets on ULVWF on endothelial surface *in vitro*; similar findings have been demonstrated *in vivo* [146]. As discussed in more detail with regards to microvascular thrombosis (Section 6.3), deficiency of ADAMTS-13 is associated with some clinical cases of severe thrombosis, including thrombotic thrombocytopenic purpura [147], and severe forms of infections [148,149]. Conceivably, ADAMTS-13 and vWF may become future therapeutic targets in thrombosis associated with inflammation [150].

3.3.3   OTHER MECHANISMS

While PSGL-1 expression on leukocytes is well characterized as a mediator of leukocyte-endothelial and leukocyte-platelet interactions, some reports suggest that endothelial cells may express functional PSGL-1 [151,152]. By binding to P-selectin on the surface of activated platelets, endothelial PSGL-1 may represent another mechanism of platelet adhesion to endothelium during inflammation [151]. Further, some data suggest that platelets may also express functional PSGL-1 [153]. The physiologic role of the putative platelet PSGL-1 and of endothelial PSGL-1 on platelet-vessel wall interactions remains to be established.

Another proposed mechanism of platelet adhesion to endothelium in inflammation is via platelet GPIIb/IIIa, through its known interaction with fibrinogen [85,154]. In an experimental model of ischemia-reperfusion injury, platelet GPIIb/IIIa mediates platelet adhesion to fibrinogen deposited on the endothelial surface. In these models, fibrinogen appears to bind to endothelium via intercellular adhesion molecule-1 (ICAM-1) on the surface of inflamed endothelial cells [154,155].

Adhesive interactions of platelets with endothelial cells are increasingly recognized in inflammatory states, and they provide insight into the known links between inflammation and thrombosis. Further, adhesion of platelets to endothelium (and to leukocytes) contributes to the roles of platelets beyond their role in hemostasis and thrombosis, including their function as mediators of acute inflammation. Our knowledge of this field is evolving.

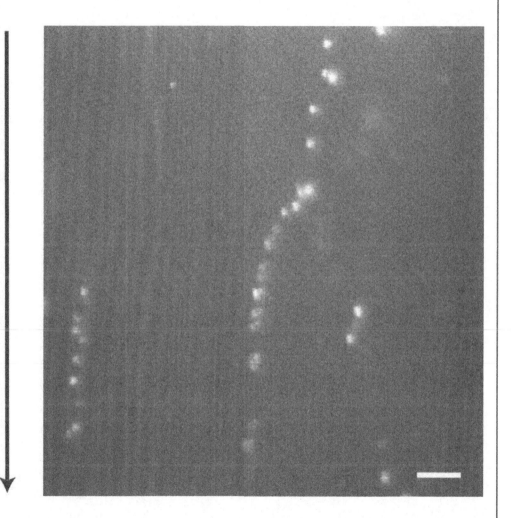

Figure 3.5: Platelet adhesion on ULVWF strings on endothelial cells in culture in a parallel-plate flow chamber, demonstrating a characteristic "bead-on-a-string" appearance (arrows). Bar = 10 μm. Figure courtesy of Jing-Fei Dong, M.D., (Baylor College of Medicine, Houston, TX).

CHAPTER 4

Platelet Aggregation

4.1   MECHANISMS OF PLATELET AGGREGATION

Aggregation involves platelet-to-platelet adhesion, and is necessary for effective hemostasis following the initial adhesion of platelets to the site of injury, described above in Chapter 3. Following adhesion, platelets are activated by a number of agonists such as adenosine diphosphate (ADP) and collagen present at the sites of vascular injury. These agonists activate platelets by binding to specific receptors on the platelet surface discussed earlier. Occupancy of these receptors leads to a series of downstream events that ultimately increases the intracytoplasmic concentration of calcium ions. The increase in platelet intracellular calcium occurs through release from intracellular stores and calcium influx through the plasma membrane [156]. Receptors coupled to G-proteins such as those to ADP, thromboxane A_2 (TXA$_2$) and thrombin, activate phospholipase Cβ (PLCβ), whereas receptors acting via the non-receptor tyrosine kinase pathways such as collagen receptor GpVI preferentially activate phospholipase Cγ (PLCγ) [83]. Activation of PLCβ or PLCγ results in the production of two second messengers: diacylglycerol (DAG) and inositol trisphosphate (IP$_3$). DAG mediates calcium influx while IP$_3$ liberates calcium from intracellular stores. In addition, calcium influx may be induced directly by certain agonists, such as ATP binding to the ligand-gated ion channel receptor, P2X1 [74].

Increased platelet free calcium concentration results in a number of structural and functional changes of the platelet. Morphologically, the platelet changes dramatically from a disc to a spiny sphere (a process called shape change). The granules in the platelet are centralized and their contents are discharged into the lumen of the open canalicular system, from which they are then released to the exterior (the release reaction). The increase in platelet calcium stimulates membrane phospholipase A_2 activity, which liberates arachidonic acid from membrane phospholipids. Arachidonic acid is converted to an intermediate product prostaglandin H_2 (PGH$_2$) by the enzyme cyclooxygenase 1 (COX-1). PGH$_2$ is further metabolized to TXA$_2$ by thromboxane synthase [117]. TXA$_2$ is a potent activator of platelets. The long membrane projections brought about by shape-change reaction allow the platelets to interact with one another to form aggregates. Shape change is mediated by the platelet cytoskeleton, composed by an organized network of microtubules and actin filaments and a number of associated proteins, linked to a variety of platelet signaling molecules [157]. Platelet shape change results in extensive reorganization of the cytoskeleton network, polymerization of actin, and myosin light chain phosphorylation [157–160]; these responses vary in a time- and stimulus-dependent manner. Examples of changes in platelet shape during activation and aggregation are depicted in Figure 4.1.

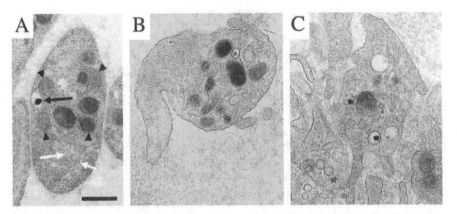

Figure 4.1: Transmission Electron microscopy images of mouse platelets illustrating various stages of activation, associated with microvascular thrombosis induced by photochemical injury. A) discoid-shape platelet revealing a dense granule with a characteristic "bull's eye" appearance (black arrow), multiple granules (arrowheads), open canalicular system and tubules (white arrows). B) platelet undergoing shape change and reorganization of granules. C) aggregate of platelets revealing extensive shape change, and paucity of granules within the aggregate. A partially activated platelet revealing dense and other granules is evident within the aggregate. Bar = 500 nm. Electron microscopy performed by Alan Burns, Ph.D. (University of Houston, Houston, TX).

A main adhesion molecule involved in platelet aggregation is the membrane protein, GPIIb/IIIa complex. GPIIb/IIIa is an integrin receptor present at high density on platelets, both on the plasma membrane and on α-granules [52]. It exists as an inactive form in resting platelets. Platelet activation by almost all agonists induces conformational changes ('inside-out signaling') of GPIIb/IIIa, which becomes competent to bind soluble plasma fibrinogen. In turn, ligand binding of GPIIb/IIIa results in conformational changes directed to the cytoplasm ('outside-in signaling'). The precise sequence of events leading to these signaling events has not been fully elucidated [53, 161]. The roles of receptor clustering, phosphorylation and association with cytoskeletal and other cytoplasmic molecules in inducing GPIIb/IIIa conformational changes are not totally delineated. Nevertheless, the receptor-bound fibrinogen acts as a bridge between two GPIIb/IIIa molecules on adjacent platelets [83]. This is the final common pathway of platelet aggregation induced by platelet chemical agonists. However, vWF substitutes for fibrinogen as a bridge molecule between GPIIb/IIIa for platelet aggregation induced by high shear conditions, although platelet aggregation under lower shear is mediated by fibrinogen binding to GPIIb/IIIa [162].

Although GPIIb/IIIa is the most widely studied mediator of bridging platelets to each other and stabilizing thrombi, other molecules have been proposed recently to mediate these responses. These include junctional adhesion molecules (JAMs), SLAM (signaling lymphocyte activation molecule) family proteins, and CD40 ligand [163–165]. The relative roles of these mechanisms in platelet aggregation are yet to be defined clearly.

Activated platelets recruit additional platelets to the growing hemostatic plug by several feedback amplification loops: they release platelet agonists (such as ADP and serotonin stored in the α-granules) and they synthesize de novo proaggregatory TXA_2. Release of ADP and TXA_2 synthesis consolidate the initial hemostatic plug by promoting the participation of other platelets in the hemostatic plug formed at sites of vascular injury. Finally, platelets also play a dominant role in secondary hemostasis by providing a highly effective catalytic surface for activation of the coagulation cascade, as discussed below in Chapter 5. When platelets are activated, negatively charged phospholipids move from the inner leaflet of the membrane bilayer to the to the outer leaflet. The transbilayer movement of anionic phospholipids is associated with blebbing and release of procoagulant vesicles rich in anionic phospholipids. Both activated platelets and the micro-vesicles provide binding sites for enzymes and cofactors of the coagulation system, which then efficiently generate thrombin, itself a potent platelet agonist.

4.2   MONITORING OF PLATELET AGGREGATION

4.2.1   EX VIVO MONITORING: PLATELET AGGREGOMETRY

Traditional approaches to monitor platelet aggregation involve exposure of platelets in suspension to a variety of stimuli *ex vivo*, a technique known as platelet aggregometry. Agonists used commonly include adenosine diphosphate (ADP), collagen, thrombin, and thromboxane A_2, among others [166]. Studies are performed on either platelet-rich plasma or whole blood; platelets are maintained in suspension by stirring. Following exposure to an agonist, formation of platelet aggregates results in an increase in light transmission through the sample; the kinetics of the responses and maximal aggregation provide quantitative assessment of platelet aggregation. Figure 4.2 illustrates aggregation response of platelets *ex vivo* in response to ADP. Platelet aggregometry may provide relevant information of platelet function abnormalities in some selected clinical conditions, though this technique is used more frequently experimentally than clinically.

4.2.2   IN VIVO MONITORING OF PLATELET AGGREGATION

While platelet aggregometry allows for assessment of platelet aggregation kinetics under carefully controlled experimental conditions (agonist dose, platelet counts, temperature, etc.), it may not reflect the complexities involved in platelet aggregation *in vivo*. A variety of intravital video microscopy approaches have been used to monitor platelet aggregation during thrombus formation *in vivo*, these are reviewed in detail elsewhere [134]. These techniques typically involve an injury to microvascular walls, for example by micropuncture, electrical stimulation, laser, chemical, or photochemical injury [86, 134, 167–169]. The nature of vascular injury, as well as the vessel type may determine the molecular mechanisms responsible for platelet recruitment in the individual models. In some models (e.g., micropuncture, chemical stimulation) platelet adhesion occurs at sites of endothelial denuda-

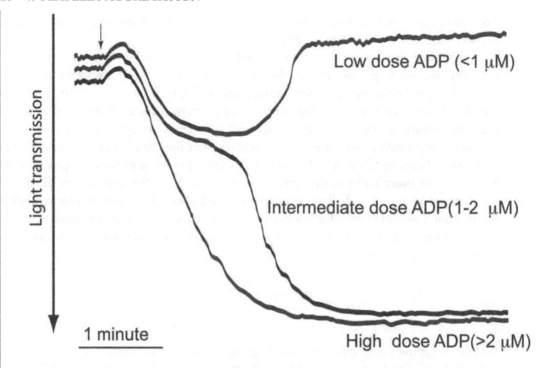

Figure 4.2: Platelet aggregometry tracing of human platelets in response to ADP. Low-dose exposure results in reversible aggregation, evident as a transient increase in light transmission. Intermediate dose results in two "waves" of aggregation, whereas high-dose exposure induces a single, irreversible wave of aggregation.

tion and reflects the mechanisms of platelet adhesion to the subendothelial matrix outlined earlier. In others, platelet adhesion is evident without overt endothelial denudation [86,170]. Vascular injury results in platelet adhesion, which may progress to formation of an occlusive thrombus, as illustrated in Figure 4.3. The kinetics of platelet adhesion and aggregation may be monitored in real-time with these techniques, and they have provided important novel observations of the mechanisms mediating platelet recruitment *in vivo*. These approaches also illustrate the redundancy of many mechanisms responsible for platelet recruitment. For example, mice lacking both vWF and fibrinogen are able to form occlusive thrombi following injury, albeit with marked delay in responses [171]. While intravital microscopy to visualize thrombus formation is not a new technique (e.g., Bizzozero used it in the late 19th century [2]), advances in image acquisition and processing techniques, molecular biology and genetic models of disease have expanded the recent interest in this approach to study interactions of platelets with vascular walls.

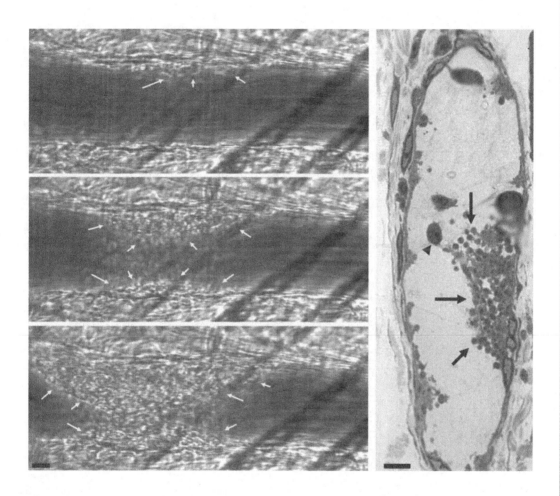

Figure 4.3: Platelet adhesion and aggregation *in vivo* in a mouse model of endothelial injury induced by photochemical stimulation. Sequential intravital microscopy images reveal progressive increase in platelet aggregates (arrows) within an injured cremaster venule; right panel reveals a cross-sectional image of an excised aggregate composed mainly of platelets (arrows) with a neutrophil evident on the periphery of the thrombus (arrowhead). Bar = 10 μm.

CHAPTER 5

Platelet Recruitment and Blood Coagulation

5.1   ROLE OF PLATELETS

In addition to their role in primary hemostasis, activated platelets provide an efficient catalytic surface for the assembly of the enzyme complexes of the blood coagulation system, also known as secondary hemostasis. The classic description of coagulation involved a cascade model consisting of two distinct pathways: the extrinsic, or tissue factor pathway and the intrinsic pathway. These are now viewed in terms of overlapping phases of initiation, amplification and propagation (Figure 5.1). These pathways have been reviewed in detail elsewhere [172–174]; we will describe them briefly and focus on the interactions between platelets and blood coagulation.

Tissue factor binds factor VIIa, which exists in low levels in the blood, and this interaction converts more factor VII to VIIa autocatalytically. More importantly, the tissue factor-VIIa complex formed activates both factor IX and factor X. Factor IXa, in the presence of factor VIIIa, catalyzes the generation of more Xa, hence amplifying this pathway. Furthermore, factor Xa can also activate factor VII to VIIa. Tissue factor pathway inhibitor (TFPI), a multivalent, plasma protease inhibitor inhibits activated factor Xa, in a factor VIIa-dependent manner providing a feedback inhibition of the tissue factor pathway. Factor Xa, in the presence of Va and Ca^{2+} catalyzes the conversion of prothrombin to thrombin on anionic phospholipid surface. Thrombin converts fibrinogen to fibrin in a multiple-step reaction, which eventually leads to formation of cross-linked and insoluble interconnecting networks of strands. In addition, thrombin activates coagulation factors V, VIII and IX to generate active forms of Va, VIIIa and IXa. Thrombin is also key mediator of platelet activation, release reaction and aggregation. Its action on platelets produces a highly efficient catalytic surface for further generation of thrombin. The coagulation system consists of a number of serine proteases, cofactors, calcium, and cell membrane components, and their reactions are frequently illustrated as simple sequential events. However, they represent highly complex interactions, subject to regulation at a number of levels.

The characteristics of the procoagulant activity on the platelet surface resemble those of synthetic phospholipid surfaces. To be active in coagulation, the phospholipid surface requires a net negative charge (provided by phosphatidylserine, phosphatidylinositol or phosphatidic acid), an optimal degree of unsaturation of the acyl chains, and an appropriate size. The most optimal procoagulant activity is observed when the phospholipid is in the micellar form with an anionic phospholipid concentration of about 20–30%. Phospholipid surfaces accelerate two distinct reactions

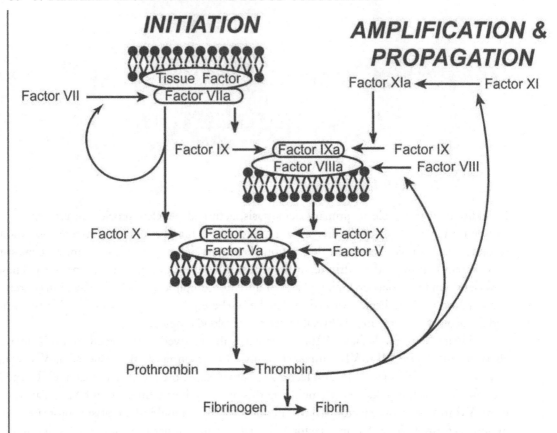

Figure 5.1: Simplified model of the major enzymatic processes of the coagulation cascade. In this model, coagulation is initiated by binding of tissue factor to factor VIIa; this complex activates Factor IX and Factor X, and converts more Factor VII to VIIa. Factor Xa, in the presence of Va and calcium catalyzes the conversion of prothrombin to thrombin. Thrombin activates these pathways at multiple levels as shown. The role of membrane phospholipids in various steps is depicted; see text for details.

in the coagulation cascade, activation of factor X by factor IXa (in the presence of factor VIIIa and Ca^{2+}) and activation of prothrombin by factor Xa (in the presence of factor Va and Ca^{2+}), by providing sites for the assembly of enzyme substrate complexes [175].

In resting platelets, phosphatidylserine and other anionic phospholipids are located on the inner aspect of the membrane bilayer [176]. Following platelet activation with thrombin, collagen, or shear stress, phosphatidylserine moves from the inner to the outer leaflet of platelet plasma membrane. This movement is associated with an increase in the activation of prothrombin and factor X [177] and with the appearance of high-affinity binding sites for factors Va and VIIIa.

The importance of the exposure of anionic phospholipid for hemostasis *in vivo* is exemplified by Scott syndrome, a rare bleeding disorder first described in 1979 by Weiss et al. as an isolated deficiency of platelet procoagulant activity [178]. The patient had a bleeding disorder, including excessive postoperative bleeding and spontaneous retroperitoneal hematomas. Her platelets aggregated normally to all agonists tested but failed to provide procoagulant activity. In a series of subsequent studies, it was shown that her platelets had a reduced number of binding sites for factor Va and VIIIa and did not promote prothrombin or factor X activation. Furthermore, following platelet activation with thrombin and collagen, there was a marked decrease in the exposure of anionic phospholipid at the platelet surface as compared with normal platelet [179]. The clinical features of this patient illustrate the importance of platelet procoagulant activity in secondary hemostasis.

The transbilayer movement of anionic phospholipid from the inner leaflet to the outer leaflet requires increases in intraplatelet Ca^{2++} and a putative enzyme named scramblase. Externalization of anionic phospholipid in platelets is accompanied by the generation of phosphatidylserine-rich microvesicles, which as far back as 1967, were shown to account for the clot-promoting activity of plasma [180]. By freeze-fracture electron microscopy they were shown to possess bilayer structure with intramembranous particles [181]. These microvesicles also contain platelet cytoskeletal proteins and platelet membrane glycoproteins Ib, IIb, IIIa and IV. The discovery of Sims et al. that microvesiculation is also defective in Scott Syndrome suggested that microvesicles and anionic phospholipid exposure are linked events and that failure to produce microvesicles may contribute to the hemostatic defect in Scott Syndrome [182].

Several findings suggest that, in addition to its role in normal hemostasis, platelet microvesiculation may contribute to the prothrombotic tendencies observed in several diseases. Platelet-derived microvesicles have been detected in the circulation in patients with disseminated intravascular coagulation [183], heparin-induced thrombocytopenia [184], the antiphospholipid antibody syndrome [185], transient ischemic attacks [186], and thrombotic thrombocytopenic purpura [187], conditions associated with either arterial, venous, and/or microvascular thrombosis. These associations suggest that, while they may be necessary for normal hemostasis, elevated microvesicle concentrations could predispose to thrombosis. Thus, conditions that increase the production or decrease the clearance of microvesicles are expected to increase the incidence of thrombosis. More recently, in addition to their hemostatic role, platelet-derived microvesicles were shown to stimulate hematopoietic cells [188] and to transfer platelet-specific receptors to the surface of other cells [189]. Microvesicles localize to sites of blood vessel damage [190] and they are incorporated to a growing thrombus [191]. In a mouse model of hemophilia, generation of microvesicles through an interaction with soluble P-selectin and PSGL-1 significantly improved the kinetics of fibrin formation in mice and normalized the prolonged tail-bleeding time [191].

Recent findings indicate that in addition to providing anionic phospholipid for prothrombin and factor X activation, microvesicles may have a major role in the initiation of thrombosis via the tissue factor pathway. These data also reveal that microvesicles relevant for thrombosis are derived from various cell types. The traditional concept of hemostasis has been that blood clotting is induced by tissue factor, a cell surface glycoprotein present on most tissues, which is derived from extravascular tissue following vessel wall injury [192]. Several studies have shown that tissue factor also circulates in the blood under normal conditions associated with cell-derived membrane microvesicles [193]. Tissue factor-bearing microvesicles are believed to arise from cells of the monocyte/macrophage lineage [194]; the role of leukocyte-derived tissue factor is discussed in greater detail in Section 5.2. The microvesicles bind activated platelets in thrombi through a molecular bridge between P-selectin glycoprotein ligand-1 (PSGL-1) on microvesicles and P-selectin on platelets. These microvesicles selectively enriched in both tissue factor and PSGL-1 fuse with activated platelets, transferring tissue factor to the platelet membrane [194]. Failure of this hemostatic mechanism may explain the ability of agents that block the PSGL-1–P-selectin interaction to significantly inhibit experimental thrombosis [195]. The role of tissue factor-bearing microvesicles in normal hemostasis is an active area of investigation.

5.2   ROLE OF PLATELET-LEUKOCYTE INTERACTIONS

Leukocytes are key mediators in the inflammatory response, and interactions between leukocytes and platelets are increasingly recognized as relevant for inflammation and thrombosis [196]. Figure 5.2 depicts several proposed mechanisms by which platelet-leukocyte interactions contribute to thrombosis.

The role of leukocytes in promoting platelet adhesion to endothelium was reviewed in Section 3.3; in addition, leukocyte-platelet interactions contribute to activation of the coagulation cascade via tissue factor-dependent pathways. While tissue factor antigen has been measured in normal plasma, it was assumed to be present in an inactive, or encrypted, form. However, a report by Giesen et al. [193] challenged this notion and prompted a re-evaluation of the role of blood-borne tissue factor in thrombosis. Those authors demonstrated that perfusion of human blood over pig arterial media (which had no detectable tissue factor) and over glass slides coated with collagen, resulted in formation of thrombi that stained intensely for tissue factor. Because the perfusion of blood was very brief (5 minutes), the authors proposed that blood-borne tissue factor mediated propagation of thrombi at sites of vascular injury. In these experiments, tissue factor was present on vesicles, which stained positively for CD18, a leukocyte marker, suggesting a leukocyte origin for these vesicles. Based on these findings, leukocyte-derived, tissue factor-bearing microvesicles are suggested to play a role in hemostasis and thrombosis. Recent data reveal that microvesicles derived from monocytes, originating from cholesterol-enriched membrane microdomains known as lipid rafts, can fuse with the membrane of activated platelets, via a mechanism involving P-selectin–PSGL-1-interactions [197]. These findings were proposed as a mechanism to explain limiting of coagulation to the sites of vascular injury, where activated platelets accumulate.

While resting monocytes contain minimal tissue factor, its synthesis is enhanced by a number of inflammatory mediators, including endotoxin, interleukin-1β, antigen–antibody complexes, tumor necrosis factor-α (TNF-α), platelet membranes, C-reactive protein, reactive oxygen species, and complement factor 5a [198]. In addition to synthesizing tissue factor, activated monocytes can

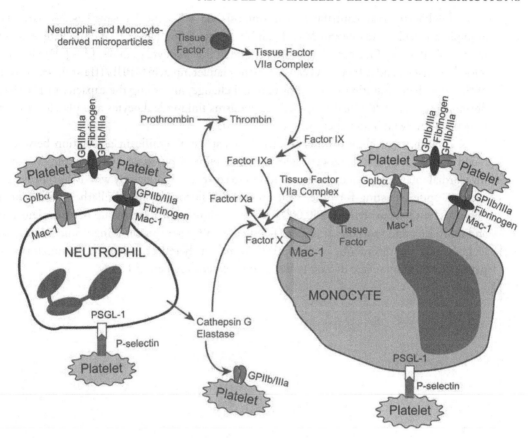

Figure 5.2: Schematic of interactions between leukocytes (neutrophil on left, monocyte on right), and platelets in activation of coagulation. The figure depicts three of the various reported mechanisms involved in platelet-leukocyte adhesion (mediated by platelet GPIbα, GPIIb/IIIa, and P-selectin). Tissue factor is also depicted as a link between leukocytes and coagulation, with tissue factor released from monocytes as well as tissue-factor-bearing microparticles derived from leukocytes. The figure also illustrates the role of leukocyte cathepsin G and elastase in activation of Factor X and platelet GPIIb/IIIa. See text for details.

activate, or decrypt, tissue factor. Like many other cells, stimulated monocytes can release microvesicles [199], though the precise mechanism of this process is not fully understood. Microvesiculation is associated with transbilayer movement of anionic phospholipids, from the inner to outer membrane bilayer, thus enabling decryption of tissue factor by these microvesicles. In addition to monocytes, neutrophils may also express tissue factor, either by de novo synthesis or via uptake of tissue factor-containing vesicles from plasma.

Leukocytes may contribute to thrombosis via other mechanisms besides tissue factor; for example, the leukocyte integrin Mac-1 can bind coagulation factor X, and mediate its activation by release of cathepsin G, a serine protease contained in leukocyte granules [200]. Further, neutrophil release of elastase and cathepsin G can cleave the platelet integrin GPIIb/IIIa at the carboxyl terminus of the α_{IIb} chain, resulting in a conformational change, increasing the capacity of platelets to bind fibrinogen [201]. Additional proposed mechanisms linking leukocytes and platelets to thrombosis have been reviewed in detail elsewhere [196,202].

A number of clinical observations demonstrate a significant association between elevated blood leukocyte count (leukocytosis) and worse clinical outcome. For example, in patients with myocardial infarction, leukocytosis was found to correlate significantly with recurrence of a coronary event, despite adjusting for other well-known risk factors [203]. Similarly, in a recent review of published studies involving >350,000 patients, a significant relationship between leukocyte count and morbidity and mortality was identified [204]. Whether these findings indicate a causal role for leukocytes in the thrombotic complications, or primarily reflect a greater inflammatory response in patients with more severe disease remains to be determined conclusively.

CHAPTER 6

Arterial, Venous, and Microvascular Hemostasis/Thrombosis

While hemostasis represents a physiological response to prevent bleeding, the term thrombosis typically refers to the pathologic formation of a thrombus (clot). This may result in severe consequences, due to reduction or cessation of blood flow to a tissue by the thrombus itself, or by rupture and release of thrombi (known as embolization). Thrombosis contributes to morbidity and mortality in common clinical diseases like myocardial infarction, stroke, deep venous thrombosis, and cancer, among many others. Since these disorders represent the most common causes of death [205], thrombosis is a major health and economic burden. Clinical and experimental thrombosis may occur throughout the vascular tree; while they share some fundamental features among the various vessel types, certain differences in pathogenesis and molecular mechanisms are evident [206–209]. A number of clinical risk factors for development of thrombosis have been identified [210, 211]; these are outlined in Table 6.1.

6.1 VENOUS THROMBOSIS

The pathophysiology of venous thrombosis is traditionally attributed to the experiments performed by Rudolph Virchow in the mid 19th century, in which he described that the consequences of thrombosis in dog pulmonary arteries could be grouped according to irritation of the blood vessel and its surroundings, to blood coagulation, and to interruption of blood flow [212]. Those observations formed the basis of "Virchow's triad" of endothelial injury, hypercoagulability and stasis, as mechanisms predisposing to formation of venous thrombosis. Venous thrombosis is a common clinical entity, associated with a number of acquired and intrinsic risk factors, including cancer, surgery, indwelling catheter use, stroke, medications, inherited hypercoagulable states, and others [211]. The relative contribution of the factors of Virchow's triad varies according to the type of venous thrombosis, and between venous and arterial thrombi. These will be discussed individually.

6.1.1 ENDOTHELIAL INJURY

The role of endothelial injury in most clinical cases of venous thrombosis is relatively unclear. Venous thrombosis occurs frequently in the veins of the lower extremities, particularly in the pockets

Table 6.1: Selected Risk Factors for Thrombosis.

Venous

 Inherited

  Antithrombin III deficiency

  Factor V Leiden

  Protein C deficiency

  Protein S deficiency

  Prothrombin gene mutation

  Fibrinolytic defects

 Acquired

  Stasis due to:

   Prolonged immobilization

   Post-operative state

   Pregnancy

  Cancer

  Nephrotic syndrome

  Myeloproliferative disorders

  Antiphospholipid antibodies

  Inflammatory bowel disease

Arterial

 Diseases of the arterial wall:

  Atherosclerosis, vasculitis,

  Diabetes mellitus, hypertension

 Platelet hyperactivity:

  Heparin-induced

  thrombocytopenia/thrombosis (HITT)

  Myeloproliferative syndrome

 Antiphospholipid antibody

 Hyperhomocysteinemia

 Smoking

 Oral contraceptives

of venous valves, which serve to direct flow against gravity. In a classic study, Sevitt [213] reported histologic findings of 50 thrombi of femoral vein valves obtained at autopsy. The thrombi consisted mainly of fibrin and varying degrees of platelets, but there was no significant evidence of damage to the vascular intima; the endothelium beneath the thrombi appeared normal. These findings suggest that overt damage to endothelium may not contribute significantly to the common entity of deep venous thrombosis. More subtle forms of endothelial injury, without overt denudation, have been proposed to contribute to thrombosis in this entity [214]. One potential stimulus for endothelial injury is hypoxia, which has been demonstrated to occur in the pockets of venous valves [215], and may result in increased expression of P-selectin on endothelial cells [216]. As outlined above in Chapter 3, P-selectin may contribute to thrombosis by various mechanisms including promoting platelet-endothelial and platelet-leukocyte-endothelial interactions. Endothelial P-selectin surface expression is associated with a variety of inflammatory stimuli, and local inflammation has also been postulated to contribute to the initiation of deep venous thrombosis [217]. The association between inflammation and venous thrombosis is illustrated by the clinical use of the term "thrombophlebitis", or inflammation of a vein related to a thrombus [218]. Inflammation has also been suggested to mediate the contribution of stasis to venous thrombosis as outlined in the next section.

   Although endothelial denudation was not detected in patients with deep vein thrombosis of the lower extremities [213], denudation may contribute to some cases of venous thrombosis, such as those associated with the use of indwelling central venous catheters [219]. Ultrastructural studies on animal models of catheter-associated thrombosis, using catheters analogous to those used clinically, demonstrate significant endothelial denudation [220]. Of interest, an association between infection and thrombosis has been well established in patients with catheter-related thrombosis [221], suggesting a role for inflammation in this entity.

6.1.2   HYPERCOAGULABILITY

The term "hypercoagulable state" is used to denote conditions that favors a procoagulant state due to imbalances in the hemostatic mechanisms, resulting in an unusual tendency toward thrombosis [210]. The changes in the hemostatic factors can often be used to predict the risk of future vascular events. The activation of coagulation factors plays a major role in venous thrombosis by concentrating these activated factors in regions of reduced flow, such as the valve pockets. Consequently, inherited defects in the anticoagulant mechanisms such as antithrombin deficiency, the protein C pathways and fibrinolytic pathways play a major role in venous thrombosis [210]. Furthermore, activation of the coagulation cascade due to release of tissue factor from damaged tissues, tumors, or cytokine stimulation also increases the risk of venous thrombosis. Stasis accentuates the local concentration of the activated coagulation factors at areas of vascular injury as discussed below.

6.1.3   STASIS

An association between stasis and venous thrombosis has long been recognized based on a number of clinical observations. In a classic study of patients with stroke and paralysis or weakness of one half of the body (hemiplegia or hemiparesis, respectively), 53% developed venous thrombosis in the paralyzed limb, whereas only 7% developed thrombosis in the non-paralyzed limb. A number of other conditions resulting in hospitalization, such as the postoperative state, are well known risk factors of venous thrombosis, particularly with prolonged bed rest [222]. Similarly, patients with factures, immobilization and orthopedic surgery are at especially high risk [223], and prolonged immobility during long-haul air flights is increasingly associated with development of venous thrombosis [224]. Although stasis clearly predisposes to development of venous thrombi, it is unclear whether stasis alone, in the absent of other components of Virchow's triad, is sufficient to initiate venous thrombosis [209]. Animal models of venous thrombosis associated with stasis typically require concomitant forms of endothelial injury such as vessel ligation or vascular injury [225,226]. Similarly, some clinical data failed to demonstrate independent effects of bed rest per se, on venous thrombosis after controlling for other clinical conditions associated with thrombosis [227]. A potential mechanism by which stasis predisposes to venous thrombosis is by inducing local hypoxia and stimulating endothelial release of P-selectin, as discussed above. In addition to P-selectin, hypoxia-induced exocytosis of Weibel-Palade bodies results in increased release of vWF [228], which may promote platelet recruitment by the mechanisms outlined previously. Hypoxia-induced stimulation of tissue factor synthesis by monocytes has also been postulated as another mechanism linking hypoxia and thrombosis [229].

6.1.4   COEXISTENCE OF VIRCHOW'S TRIAD COMPONENTS: CANCER AND THROMBOSIS

In a number of clinical entities, more than one component of Virchow's triad may contribute to the pathogenesis of thrombosis. A prominent example of this is evident in thrombosis associated with cancer [230]. Patients with cancer have a nearly 7-fold increased risk of venous thrombosis as compared to patients without malignancy, and approximately 20% of new cases of venous thrombosis are associated with cancer [231–233]. Cancer may contribute to a hypercoagulable state; for example, cancer cells express tissue factor and can release tissue factor-bearing microparticles [234]. Of interest, the degree of tissue factor expression on some tumors has been correlated with greater risk of development of venous thrombosis [234,235]. Other proposed factors derived from cancer leading to a hypercoagulable state include cancer procoagulant, cytokines, and fibrinolytic substances [236]. In addition to hypercoagulability, endothelial injury has been suggested to contribute to venous thrombosis in cancer. In certain tumors, direct extension of cancer cells into blood vessels may result in formation of thrombi [237]. In addition, indirect endothelial activation via cytokines may promote thrombosis [236], by similar mechanisms as those outlined under platelet-endothelial adhesion in Section 3.3. Further, cancer-derived microparticles may mediate endothelial injury; recent data demonstrate incorporation of these microparticles at the sites of endothelial injury in a mouse model of thrombosis [238]. Cancer may also promote thrombosis by contributing to stasis; for example as a result of vascular compression by the tumor or enlarged lymph nodes [239], or by the associated reduced mobility [240]. Finally, catheter-associated thrombosis are common in patients with cancer, due to the frequent use of these devices in this patient population [241].

6.2   ARTERIAL THROMBOSIS

Consequences of arterial thrombosis such as myocardial infarction and stroke are the most common causes of morbidity and mortality in middle-aged Americans. Though the clinical manifestation of myocardial infarction and strokes are different, they are the result of the same pathogenic process, formation of a thrombus over an underlying atherosclerotic plaque in the setting of high flow and high shear arterial circulation [242]. In most cases, the thrombus overlies a ruptured plaque or an intact plaque with superficial endothelial erosion. In recent years, it has been recognized that plaque composition rather than plaque size or severity of stenosis is important for plaque rupture and subsequent thrombosis [243] . Exposure of blood to the procoagulant materials in the ruptured plaque promotes thrombosis. Catalytically active tissue factor is present in the atherosclerotic plaque and seems to play a major role in the initialization of thrombosis following rupture [244, 245]. Under arterial shear stresses, only platelets are capable of adhesion to the damaged vessel wall. Several adhesion molecules and platelet agonists are present in the plaque such as collagen, and oxidized lipids [246]. In contrast to venous thrombosis, activation of coagulation factors does not appear to play a major role in arterial thrombosis as these factors are likely to be removed by the high flow in the arterial system. Vessel wall damage due to atherosclerosis, hypertension, or vascular anomalies is a major risk factor for arterial thrombosis, by inducing turbulence and altered blood flow, which allows platelet adhesion. Consequently, hyperactivity of platelets also plays a role in the pathogenesis. Antiplatelet therapy such as aspirin is used very successfully to prevent vascular events in arterial thrombosis while they are of limited value in preventing venous thrombosis.

6.3   MICROVASCULAR THROMBOSIS

Thrombosis of large arteries and veins typically receive the greatest attention clinically and experimentally, likely due to the health and economic impact of those disorders. Thrombosis may also occur within the microcirculation, which represents the largest proportion of the surface area of the vasculature. Microvascular thrombi have been demonstrated in a number of severe clinical diseases, including thrombotic thrombocytopenic purpura, sepsis, disseminated intravascular coagulation, and antiphospholipid syndrome among others [247–250]. The ultrastructure of thrombi in these diseases varies widely, ranging from platelet-rich "white" thrombi to fibrin- and erythrocyte-rich "red" thrombi. Microvascular thrombosis has been demonstrated in various organs and various vessel types in those disorders, though their tissue and vessel distribution vary among those entities. Microvessels consist of arterioles, capillaries and venules and demonstrate considerable heterogeneity in vascular wall structure, function, and endothelial interactions with blood constituents. Figure 6.1 illustrates a few of the prominent differences between arterioles and venules: endothelial cell morphology, leukocyte-endothelial interactions, vascular smooth muscle content, and endothelial von Willebrand factor expression.

Of interest, in addition to the marked structural differences between arterioles and venules, these vessels demonstrate significant differences in their responses to thrombosis induced by various

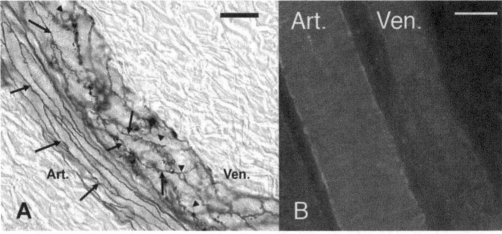

Figure 6.1: Example of several structural differences between arterioles and venules. A) Silver-stained microvessels of the rat mesentery. The endothelial cell borders (arrows) reveal long spindle-shaped cells in arterioles (Art.) and polygonal cells in venules (Ven.). Adherent leukocytes (arrowheads) are evident only on venules. B) Immunofluorescence of mouse cremaster microvessels demonstrating vascular smooth muscle limited to the arteriole (stained with alpha smooth muscle alpha actin, (green) and considerably greater von Willebrand factor expression (stained red) in the venule. Panel B from reference [92], with permission.

forms of endothelial injury, as determined by intravital microscopy-based models. These include a predisposition of venules to microvascular thrombosis as well as significant differences in kinetics of thrombus formation and embolization between venules and arterioles [86,134,167]. These studies also suggest differences in endogenous mechanisms preventing thrombosis and embolization among venules and arterioles. For example, data derived from micropuncture experiments demonstrate that prostacyclin-induced inhibition of thromboembolism predominated in arterioles, while nitric oxide-induced inhibition predominated in venules [109,110,251,252]. Similarly, the influence of pathologic stimuli on experimental microvascular thrombosis differs among these vessel types, while endotoxemia promotes photochemically-induced microvascular thrombosis predominantly in venules, experimental colitis promotes thrombosis mainly on arterioles [92,138,253].

The mechanisms accounting for the differences in microvascular thrombotic responses between venules and arterioles are not fully understood. Differences in wall shear rate (much higher in arterioles) and leukocyte-endothelial interactions (which occur mainly in venules) have been suggested [134,254], though experimental evidence has failed to support them consistently [86,255]. Vascular-specific differences in nitric oxide, prostacyclin, or vWF may represent additional mechanisms contributing to the differential responses [92,109,110], and synergistic effects between these various candidates are yet to be defined.

While the mechanisms for microvascular thrombosis in each of the above-mentioned clinical disorders remain to be elucidated, a role for vWF (particularly ULVWF) is evident in certain conditions. For example, patients with a familial form of thrombotic thrombocytopenic purpura have a deficiency in ADAMTS-13, reduced cleavage of ULVWF and evidence of increased plasma levels of the large adhesive ULVWF multimers [256]. Platelet adhesion to ULVWF in the absence of ADAMTS-13 has been demonstrated both *in vitro* (see Figure 3.5) and *in vivo* [145, 146]. Similarly, some patients with severe forms of sepsis, a systemic inflammatory response to an infection, have been shown to have a secondary form of ADAMTS-13 deficiency and evidence of circulating ULVWF [148, 149]. The reduced ADAMTS-13 may contribute to microvascular thrombosis accompanying severe sepsis and disseminated intravascular coagulation [148, 149]. The increasing interest in intravital microscopy-based studies is expected to broaden our understanding of the mechanisms of microvascular thrombosis in relevant models of human diseases.

CHAPTER 7

Summary

The interactions between platelets and vascular walls mediate the physiologic process of hemostasis as well as the pathologic entity of thrombosis. These phenomena demonstrate key differences among vascular beds, and between macro- and microvessels. As outlined in this review, a large number of aspects of hemostasis and thrombosis remain as areas of active investigation. A few selected examples include the links between inflammation and thrombosis, the role of microparticles in thrombosis, mechanisms of cancer-associated thrombosis, the role of the glycocalyx as an endogenous barrier to thrombosis, development of novel antithrombotic agents, and understanding the regulation of multiple redundant mechanisms involved in hemostasis and thrombosis. Advances in molecular biology, genetics, mouse models of human disease, and imaging of thrombosis *in vivo*, among others, have provided novel tools to address these important unresolved questions. Given the major health care and economic impact of thrombosis, advances in this important field are expected to result in novel therapeutic approaches for patients with these significant clinical problems.

Bibliography

[1] Chen J and Lopez JA. Interactions of platelets with subendothelium and endothelium. Microcirculation 12, 2005. DOI: 10.1080/10739680590925484 1, 14

[2] Bizzozero J. Ueber einen neuen formbestandtheil des blutes und dessen rolle bei der thrombose und der blutgerinnung. Virchows Arch Pathol Anat Physiol Klinishe Medicine 90: 261–332, 1882. DOI: 10.1007/BF01931360 3, 26

[3] Hanson SR and Slichter SJ. Platelet kinetics in patients with bone marrow hypoplasia: evidence for a fixed platelet requirement. Blood 66: 1105–1109, 1985. 3

[4] Spaet TH. Progress in Hemostasis and Thrombosis. Volume 2. New York: Grune & Stratton, 1974. 3

[5] White JG. Electron opaque structures in human platelets: which are or are not dense bodies? Platelets 19: 455–466, 2008. DOI: 10.1080/09537100802132671 3, 4

[6] Slichter SJ. Relationship between platelet count and bleeding risk in thrombocytopenic patients. Transfus Med Rev 18: 153–167, 2004. DOI: 10.1016/j.tmrv.2004.03.003 3

[7] White JG, Krumwiede MD, Escolar G. Glycoprotein Ib is homogeneously distributed on external and internal membranes of resting platelets. Am J Pathol 155: 2127–2134, 1999. DOI: 10.1097/00000478-199903000-00001 3

[8] White JG and Clawson CC. The surface-connected canalicular system of blood platelets–a fenestrated membrane system. Am J Pathol 101: 353–364, 1980. 3

[9] Rendu F and Brohard-Bohn B. The platelet release reaction: granules' constituents, secretion and functions. Platelets 12: 261–273, 2001. DOI: 10.1080/09537100120068170 3, 5, 6

[10] Ebbeling L, Robertson C, McNicol A, Gerrard JM. Rapid ultrastructural changes in the dense tubular system following platelet activation. Blood 80: 718–723, 1992. 3

[11] Blair P and Flaumenhaft R. Platelet alpha-granules: basic biology and clinical correlates. Blood Rev 23: 177–189, 2009. DOI: 10.1016/j.blre.2009.04.001 4, 5

[12] Maynard DM, Heijnen HF, Horne MK, White JG, Gahl WA. Proteomic analysis of platelet alpha-granules using mass spectrometry. J Thromb Haemost 5: 1945–1955, 2007. DOI: 10.1111/j.1538-7836.2007.02690.x 5

[13] Italiano JE, Jr., Richardson JL, Patel-Hett S, Battinelli E, Zaslavsky A, Short S, Ryeom S, Folkman J, Klement GL. Angiogenesis is regulated by a novel mechanism: pro- and antiangiogenic proteins are organized into separate platelet alpha granules and differentially released. Blood 111: 1227–1233, 2008. 5

[14] Sehgal S and Storrie B. Evidence that differential packaging of the major platelet granule proteins von Willebrand factor and fibrinogen can support their differential release. J Thromb Haemost 5: 2009–2016, 2007. DOI: 10.1111/j.1538-7836.2007.02698.x 5

[15] Stenberg PE, Shuman MA, Levine SP, Bainton DF. Redistribution of alpha-granules and their contents in thrombin-stimulated platelets. J Cell Biol 98: 748–760, 1984. DOI: 10.1083/jcb.98.2.748 5

[16] Morgenstern E, Neumann K, Patscheke H. The exocytosis of human blood platelets. A fast freezing and freeze-substitution analysis. Eur J Cell Biol 43: 273–282, 1987. 5

[17] Flaumenhaft R. Molecular basis of platelet granule secretion. Arterioscler Thromb Vasc Biol 23: 1152–1160, 2003. DOI: 10.1161/01.ATV.0000075965.88456.48 5

[18] Lemons PP, Chen D, Bernstein AM, Bennett MK, Whiteheart SW. Regulated secretion in platelets: identification of elements of the platelet exocytosis machinery. Blood 90: 1490–1500, 1997. 5

[19] Merten M and Thiagarajan P. P-selectin in arterial thrombosis. Z Kardiol 93: 855–863, 2004. DOI: 10.1007/s00392-004-0146-5 5, 8

[20] Nurden AT and Nurden P. The gray platelet syndrome: clinical spectrum of the disease. Blood Rev 21: 21–36, 2007. DOI: 10.1016/j.blre.2005.12.003 5

[21] Chen D, Bernstein AM, Lemons PP, Whiteheart SW. Molecular mechanisms of platelet exocytosis: role of SNAP-23 and syntaxin 2 in dense core granule release. Blood 95: 921–929, 2000. 5

[22] Huizing M, Anikster Y, Gahl WA. Hermansky-Pudlak syndrome and Chediak-Higashi syndrome: disorders of vesicle formation and trafficking. Thromb Haemost 86: 233–245, 2001. 5, 6

[23] Wei ML. Hermansky-Pudlak syndrome: a disease of protein trafficking and organelle function. Pigment Cell Res 19: 19–42, 2006. DOI: 10.1111/j.1600-0749.2005.00289.x 6

[24] Li W, Rusiniak ME, Chintala S, Gautam R, Novak EK, Swank RT. Murine Hermansky-Pudlak syndrome genes: regulators of lysosome-related organelles. Bioessays 26: 616–628, 2004. DOI: 10.1002/bies.20042 6

[25] Karim MA, Nagle DL, Kandil HH, Burger J, Moore KJ, Spritz RA. Mutations in the Chediak-Higashi syndrome gene (CHS1) indicate requirement for the complete 3801 amino acid CHS protein. Hum Mol Genet 6: 1087–1089, 1997. DOI: 10.1093/hmg/6.7.1087 6

[26] Rendu F, Breton-Gorius J, Lebret M, Klebanoff C, Buriot D, Griscelli C, Levy-Toledano S, Caen JP. Evidence that abnormal platelet functions in human Chediak-Higashi syndrome are the result of a lack of dense bodies. Am J Pathol 111: 307–314, 1983. 6

[27] Ciferri S, Emiliani C, Guglielmini G, Orlacchio A, Nenci GG, Gresele P. Platelets release their lysosomal content in vivo in humans upon activation. Thromb Haemost 83: 157–164, 2000. 6

[28] Bentfeld-Barker ME and Bainton DF. Identification of primary lysosomes in human megakaryocytes and platelets. Blood 59: 472–481, 1982. 6

[29] Ren Q, Barber HK, Crawford GL, Karim ZA, Zhao C, Choi W, Wang CC, Hong W, Whiteheart SW. Endobrevin/VAMP-8 is the primary v-SNARE for the platelet release reaction. Mol Biol Cell 18: 24–33, 2007. DOI: 10.1091/mbc.E06-09-0785 6

[30] Chen D, Lemons PP, Schraw T, Whiteheart SW. Molecular mechanisms of platelet exocytosis: role of SNAP-23 and syntaxin 2 and 4 in lysosome release. Blood 96: 1782–1788, 2000. 6

[31] Silverstein RL and Febbraio M. Identification of lysosome-associated membrane protein-2 as an activation-dependent platelet surface glycoprotein. Blood 80: 1470–1475, 1992. 6

[32] Israels SJ, Gerrard JM, Jacques YV, McNicol A, Cham B, Nishibori M, Bainton DF. Platelet dense granule membranes contain both granulophysin and P-selectin (GMP-140). Blood 80: 143–152, 1992. 8

[33] Whiss PA, Andersson RG, Srinivas U. Modulation of P-selectin expression on isolated human platelets by an NO donor assessed by a novel ELISA application. J Immunol Methods 200: 135–143, 1997. DOI: 10.1016/S0022-1759(96)00198-6 8

[34] Merten M and Thiagarajan P. P-selectin expression on platelets determines size and stability of platelet aggregates. Circulation 102: 1931–1936, 2000. 8

[35] Dubois C, Panicot-Dubois L, Gainor JF, Furie BC, Furie B. Thrombin-initiated platelet activation in vivo is vWF independent during thrombus formation in a laser injury model. J Clin Invest 117: 953–960, 2007. DOI: 10.1172/JCI30537 8

[36] Padilla A, Moake JL, Bernardo A, Ball C, Wang Y, Arya M, Nolasco L, Turner N, Berndt MC, Anvari B, Lopez JA, Dong JF. P-selectin anchors newly released ultralarge von Willebrand factor multimers to the endothelial cell surface. Blood 103: 2150–2156, 2004. DOI: 10.1182/blood-2003-08-2956 8, 20

[37] Romo GM, Dong JF, Schade AJ, Gardiner EE, Kansas GS, Li CQ, McIntire LV, Berndt MC, Lopez JA. The glycoprotein Ib-IX-V complex is a platelet counterreceptor for P-selectin. J Exp Med 190: 803–814, 1999. DOI: 10.1084/jem.190.6.803 8

[38] Merten M, Beythien C, Gutensohn K, Kuhnl P, Meinertz T, Thiagarajan P. Sulfatides activate platelets through P-selectin and enhance platelet and platelet-leukocyte aggregation. Arterioscler Thromb Vasc Biol 25: 258–263, 2005. DOI: 10.1161/01.ATV.0000149675.83552.83 8

[39] Tailor A, Cooper D, Granger DN. Platelet-vessel wall interactions in the microcirculation. Microcirculation 12: 275–285, 2005. DOI: 10.1080/10739680590925691 8, 18, 19

[40] Andre P, Hartwell D, Hrachovinova I, Saffaripour S, Wagner DD. Pro-coagulant state resulting from high levels of soluble P-selectin in blood. Proc Natl Acad Sci USA 97: 13835–13840, 2000. DOI: 10.1073/pnas.250475997 8

[41] Andrews RK, Gardiner EE, Shen Y, Whisstock JC, Berndt MC. Glycoprotein Ib-IX-V. Int J Biochem Cell Biol 35: 1170–1174, 2003. 8

[42] Jurk K, Clemetson KJ, de Groot PG, Brodde MF, Steiner M, Savion N, Varon D, Sixma JJ, Van Aken H, Kehrel BE. Thrombospondin-1 mediates platelet adhesion at high shear via glycoprotein Ib (GPIb): an alternative/backup mechanism to von Willebrand factor. FASEB J 17: 1490–1492, 2003. DOI: 10.1096/fj.02-0830fje 8

[43] Simon DI, Chen Z, Xu H, Li CQ, Dong J, McIntire LV, Ballantyne CM, Zhang L, Furman MI, Berndt MC, Lopez JA. Platelet glycoprotein ibalpha is a counterreceptor for the leukocyte integrin Mac-1 (CD11b/CD18). J Exp Med 192: 193–204, 2000. DOI: 10.1084/jem.192.2.193 8, 19

[44] Harmon JT and Jamieson GA. The glycocalicin portion of platelet glycoprotein Ib expresses both high and moderate affinity receptor sites for thrombin. A soluble radioreceptor assay for the interaction of thrombin with platelets. J Biol Chem 261: 13224–13229, 1986. 8

[45] Weeterings C, de Groot PG, Adelmeijer J, Lisman T. The glycoprotein Ib-IX-V complex contributes to tissue factor-independent thrombin generation by recombinant factor VIIa on the activated platelet surface. Blood 112: 3227–3233, 2008. DOI: 10.1182/blood-2008-02-139113 8

[46] Bradford HN, Pixley RA, Colman RW. Human factor XII binding to the glycoprotein Ib-IX-V complex inhibits thrombin-induced platelet aggregation. J Biol Chem 275: 22756–22763, 2000. DOI: 10.1074/jbc.M002591200 8

[47] Baglia FA, Shrimpton CN, Emsley J, Kitagawa K, Ruggeri ZM, Lopez JA, Walsh PN. Factor XI interacts with the leucine-rich repeats of glycoprotein Ibalpha on the activated platelet. J Biol Chem 279: 49323–49329, 2004. DOI: 10.1074/jbc.M407889200 8

[48] Chavakis T, Santoso S, Clemetson KJ, Sachs UJ, Isordia-Salas I, Pixley RA, Nawroth PP, Colman RW, Preissner KT. High molecular weight kininogen regulates platelet-leukocyte interactions by bridging Mac-1 and glycoprotein Ib. J Biol Chem 278: 45375–45381, 2003. DOI: 10.1074/jbc.M304344200 8

[49] Pham A and Wang J. Bernard-Soulier syndrome: an inherited platelet disorder. Arch Pathol Lab Med 131: 1834–1836, 2007. 8

[50] Kunishima S, Kamiya T, Saito H. Genetic abnormalities of Bernard-Soulier syndrome. Int J Hematol 76: 319–327, 2002. DOI: 10.1007/BF02982690 8

[51] Coller BS, Peerschke EI, Scudder LE, Sullivan CA. Studies with a murine monoclonal antibody that abolishes ristocetin-induced binding of von Willebrand factor to platelets: additional evidence in support of GPIb as a platelet receptor for von Willebrand factor. Blood 61: 99–110, 1983. 9

[52] Niiya K, Hodson E, Bader R, Byers-Ward V, Koziol JA, Plow EF, Ruggeri ZM. Increased surface expression of the membrane glycoprotein IIb/IIIa complex induced by platelet activation. Relationship to the binding of fibrinogen and platelet aggregation. Blood 70: 475–483, 1987. 9, 24

[53] Ma YQ, Qin J, Plow EF. Platelet integrin alpha(IIb)beta(3): activation mechanisms. J Thromb Haemost 5: 1345–1352, 2007. DOI: 10.1111/j.1538-7836.2007.02537.x 9, 10, 24

[54] Bennett JS, Berger BW, Billings PC. The structure and function of platelet integrins. J Thromb Haemost 7 Suppl 1: 200–205, 2009. DOI: 10.1111/j.1538-7836.2009.03378.x 9, 15

[55] Bennett JS. Structure and function of the platelet integrin alphaIIbbeta3. J Clin Invest 115: 3363–3369, 2005. DOI: 10.1172/JCI26989 10

[56] Thomas D and Giugliano RP. Antiplatelet therapy in early management of non-ST-segment elevation acute coronary syndrome: the 2002 and 2007 guidelines from North America and Europe. J Cardiovasc Pharmacol 51: 425–433, 2008. DOI: 10.1097/FJC.0b013e31816a35a2 10, 12

[57] Farndale RW, Lisman T, Bihan D, Hamaia S, Smerling CS, Pugh N, Konitsiotis A, Leitinger B, de Groot PG, Jarvis GE, Raynal N. Cell-collagen interactions: the use of peptide Toolkits to investigate collagen-receptor interactions. Biochem Soc Trans 36: 241–250, 2008. DOI: 10.1042/BST0360241 10

[58] Smethurst PA, Onley DJ, Jarvis GE, O'Connor MN, Knight CG, Herr AB, Ouwehand WH, Farndale RW. Structural basis for the platelet-collagen interaction: the smallest motif within collagen that recognizes and activates platelet Glycoprotein VI contains two glycine-proline-hydroxyproline triplets. J Biol Chem 282: 1296–1304, 2007. DOI: 10.1074/jbc.M606479200 11

[59] Knight CG, Morton LF, Onley DJ, Peachey AR, Messent AJ, Smethurst PA, Tuckwell DS, Farndale RW, Barnes MJ. Identification in collagen type I of an integrin alpha2 beta1-binding site containing an essential GER sequence. J Biol Chem 273: 33287–33294, 1998. DOI: 10.1074/jbc.273.50.33287 11

[60] Guidetti GF, Bernardi B, Consonni A, Rizzo P, Gruppi C, Balduini C, Torti M. Integrin alpha2beta1 induces phosphorylation-dependent and phosphorylation-independent activation of phospholipase Cgamma2 in platelets: role of Src kinase and Rac GTPase. J Thromb Haemost 7: 1200–1206, 2009. DOI: 10.1111/j.1538-7836.2009.03444.x 11

[61] Suzuki H, Murasaki K, Kodama K, Takayama H. Intracellular localization of glycoprotein VI in human platelets and its surface expression upon activation. Br J Haematol 121: 904–912, 2003. DOI: 10.1046/j.1365-2141.2003.04373.x 11

[62] Moroi M and Jung SM. Platelet glycoprotein VI: its structure and function. Thromb Res 114: 221–233, 2004. DOI: 10.1016/j.thromres.2004.06.046 11

[63] Kim S, Mangin P, Dangelmaier C, Lillian R, Jackson SP, Daniel JL, Kunapuli SP. The role of PI 3-K{beta} in glycoprotein VI-mediated akt activation in platelets. J Biol Chem, 2009. DOI: 10.1074/jbc.M109.048553 11

[64] Gibbins J, Asselin J, Farndale R, Barnes M, Law CL, Watson SP. Tyrosine phosphorylation of the Fc receptor gamma-chain in collagen-stimulated platelets. J Biol Chem 271: 18095–18099, 1996. 11

[65] Arthur JF, Dunkley S, Andrews RK. Platelet glycoprotein VI-related clinical defects. Br J Haematol 139: 363–372, 2007. DOI: http://doi.wiley.com/10.1111/j.1365-2141.2007.06799.x 11

[66] Coughlin SR. Protease-activated receptors in vascular biology. Thromb Haemost 86: 298–307, 2001. 11

[67] Kahn ML, Nakanishi-Matsui M, Shapiro MJ, Ishihara H, Coughlin SR. Protease-activated receptors 1 and 4 mediate activation of human platelets by thrombin. J Clin Invest 103: 879–887, 1999. DOI: 10.1172/JCI6042 11

[68] Ishihara H, Zeng D, Connolly AJ, Tam C, Coughlin SR. Antibodies to protease-activated receptor 3 inhibit activation of mouse platelets by thrombin. Blood 91: 4152–4157, 1998. 11

[69] Ishihara H, Connolly AJ, Zeng D, Kahn ML, Zheng YW, Timmons C, Tram T, Coughlin SR. Protease-activated receptor 3 is a second thrombin receptor in humans. Nature 386: 502–506, 1997. DOI: 10.1038/386502a0 11

[70] Woulfe DS. Platelet G protein-coupled receptors in hemostasis and thrombosis. J Thromb Haemost 3: 2193–2200, 2005. DOI: 10.1111/j.1538-7836.2005.01338.x 11

[71] TRA-CER_Executive_and_Steering_Committees. The Thrombin Receptor Antagonist for Clinical Event Reduction in Acute Coronary Syndrome (TRA*CER) trial: study design and rationale. Am Heart J 158: 327–334 e324, 2009. 11

[72] Price MJ. Bedside evaluation of thienopyridine antiplatelet therapy. Circulation 119: 2625–2632, 2009. DOI: 10.1161/CIRCULATIONAHA.107.696732 12

[73] Hollopeter G, Jantzen HM, Vincent D, Li G, England L, Ramakrishnan V, Yang RB, Nurden P, Nurden A, Julius D, Conley PB. Identification of the platelet ADP receptor targeted by antithrombotic drugs. Nature 409: 202–207, 2001. DOI: 10.1038/35051599 12

[74] Murugappan S, Shankar H, Kunapuli SP. Platelet receptors for adenine nucleotides and thromboxane A2. Semin Thromb Hemost 30: 411–418, 2004. DOI: 10.1055/s-2004-833476 12, 23

[75] Habib A, FitzGerald GA, Maclouf J. Phosphorylation of the thromboxane receptor alpha, the predominant isoform expressed in human platelets. J Biol Chem 274: 2645–2651, 1999. DOI: 10.1074/jbc.274.5.2645 12

[76] Nakahata N. Thromboxane A2: physiology/pathophysiology, cellular signal transduction and pharmacology. Pharmacol Ther 118: 18–35, 2008. DOI: 10.1016/j.pharmthera.2008.01.001 12

[77] Catella-Lawson F, Reilly MP, Kapoor SC, Cucchiara AJ, DeMarco S, Tournier B, Vyas SN, FitzGerald GA. Cyclooxygenase inhibitors and the antiplatelet effects of aspirin. N Engl J Med 345: 1809–1817, 2001. DOI: 10.1056/NEJMoa003199 12

[78] Patrignani P, Filabozzi P, Patrono C. Selective cumulative inhibition of platelet thromboxane production by low-dose aspirin in healthy subjects. J Clin Invest 69: 1366–1372, 1982. DOI: 10.1172/JCI110576 12

[79] Bousser MG, Amarenco P, Chamorro A, Fisher M, Ford I, Fox K, Hennerici MG, Mattle HP, Rothwell PM. Rationale and design of a randomized, double-blind, parallel-group study of terutroban 30 mg/day versus aspirin 100 mg/day in stroke patients: the prevention of cerebrovascular and cardiovascular events of ischemic origin with terutroban in patients with a history of ischemic stroke or transient ischemic attack (PERFORM) study. Cerebrovasc Dis 27: 509–518, 2009. DOI: 10.1159/000212671 12

[80] Tangelder GJ, Teirlinck HC, Slaaf DW, Reneman RS. Distribution of blood platelets flowing in arterioles. Am J Physiol 248: H318–323, 1985. 13

[81] Woldhuis B, Tangelder GJ, Slaaf DW, Reneman RS. Concentration profile of blood platelets differs in arterioles and venules. Am J Physiol 262: H1217–1223, 1992. 13

[82] Fujimura Y, Titani K, Holland LZ, Russell SR, Roberts JR, Elder JH, Ruggeri ZM, Zimmerman TS. von Willebrand factor. A reduced and alkylated 52/48-kDa fragment beginning at amino acid residue 449 contains the domain interacting with platelet glycoprotein Ib. J Biol Chem 261: 381–385, 1986. 14

[83] Varga-Szabo D, Pleines I, Nieswandt B. Cell adhesion mechanisms in platelets. Arterioscler Thromb Vasc Biol 28: 403–412, 2008. DOI: 10.1161/ATVBAHA.107.150474 14, 23, 24

[84] Ruggeri ZM. The role of von Willebrand factor in thrombus formation. Thromb Res 120 Suppl 1: S5–9, 2007. DOI: 10.1016/j.thromres.2007.03.011 14

[85] Savage B, Saldivar E, Ruggeri ZM. Initiation of platelet adhesion by arrest onto fibrinogen or translocation on von Willebrand factor. Cell 84: 289–297, 1996. DOI: 10.1016/S0092-8674(00)80983-6 14, 20

[86] Rumbaut RE, Randhawa JK, Smith CW, Burns AR. Mouse cremaster venules are predisposed to light/dye-induced thrombosis independent of wall shear rate, CD18, ICAM-1, or P-selectin. Microcirculation 11: 239–247, 2004. DOI: 10.1080/10739680490425949 14, 25, 26, 40

[87] Konstantinides S, Ware J, Marchese P, Almus-Jacobs F, Loskutoff DJ, Ruggeri ZM. Distinct antithrombotic consequences of platelet glycoprotein Ibalpha and VI deficiency in a mouse model of arterial thrombosis. J Thromb Haemost 4: 2014–2021, 2006. DOI: 10.1111/j.1538-7836.2006.02086.x 14

[88] Ruggeri ZM, Orje JN, Habermann R, Federici AB, Reininger AJ. Activation-independent platelet adhesion and aggregation under elevated shear stress. Blood 108: 1903–1910, 2006. DOI: 10.1182/blood-2006-04-011551 14

[89] Mailhac A, Badimon JJ, Fallon JT, Fernandez-Ortiz A, Meyer B, Chesebro JH, Fuster V, Badimon L. Effect of an eccentric severe stenosis on fibrin(ogen) deposition on severely damaged vessel wall in arterial thrombosis. Relative contribution of fibrin(ogen) and platelets. Circulation 90: 988–996, 1994. 14

[90] Laffan M, Brown SA, Collins PW, Cumming AM, Hill FG, Keeling D, Peake IR, Pasi KJ. The diagnosis of von Willebrand disease: a guideline from the UK Haemophilia Centre Doctors' Organization. Haemophilia 10: 199–217, 2004. DOI: 10.1111/j.1365-2516.2004.00894.x 14

[91] Denis C, Methia N, Frenette PS, Rayburn H, Ullman-Cullere M, Hynes RO, Wagner DD. A mouse model of severe von Willebrand disease: defects in hemostasis and thrombosis. Proc Natl Acad Sci USA 95: 9524–9529, 1998. DOI: 10.1073/pnas.95.16.9524 14

[92] Patel KN, Soubra SH, Bellera RV, Dong JF, McMullen CA, Burns AR, Rumbaut RE. Differential role of von Willebrand factor and P-selectin on microvascular thrombosis in endotoxemia. Arterioscler Thromb Vasc Biol 28: 2225–2230, 2008. DOI: 10.1161/ATVBAHA.108.175679 14, 40

[93] Farndale RW. Collagen-induced platelet activation. Blood Cells Mol Dis 36: 162–165, 2006. DOI: 10.1016/j.bcmd.2005.12.016 14

[94] Cruz MA, Chen J, Whitelock JL, Morales LD, Lopez JA. The platelet glycoprotein Ib-von Willebrand factor interaction activates the collagen receptor alpha2beta1 to bind collagen: activation-dependent conformational change of the alpha2-I domain. Blood 105: 1986–1991, 2005. 14

[95] Sarratt KL, Chen H, Zutter MM, Santoro SA, Hammer DA, Kahn ML. GPVI and alpha2beta1 play independent critical roles during platelet adhesion and aggregate formation to collagen under flow. Blood 106: 1268–1277, 2005. DOI: 10.1182/blood-2004-11-4434 14

[96] Nieswandt B, Brakebusch C, Bergmeier W, Schulte V, Bouvard D, Mokhtari-Nejad R, Lindhout T, Heemskerk JW, Zirngibl H, Fassler R. Glycoprotein VI but not alpha2beta1 integrin is essential for platelet interaction with collagen. Embo J 20: 2120–2130, 2001. DOI: 10.1093/emboj/20.9.2120 14

[97] Jennings LK. Role of platelets in atherothrombosis. Am J Cardiol 103: 4A-10A, 2009. DOI: 10.1016/j.amjcard.2008.11.017 15

[98] Palmer RM, Ferrige AG, Moncada S. Nitric oxide release accounts for the biological activity of endothelium-derived relaxing factor. Nature 327: 524–526, 1987. DOI: 10.1038/327524a0 15

[99] Furchgott RF and Zawadzki JV. The obligatory role of endothelial cells in the relaxation of arterial smooth muscle by acetylcholine. Nature 288: 373–376, 1980. DOI: 10.1038/288373a0 15

[100] Moncada S and Higgs EA. The discovery of nitric oxide and its role in vascular biology. Br J Pharmacol 147 Suppl 1: S193–201, 2006. DOI: 10.1038/sj.bjp.0706458 15

[101] Dudzinski DM, Igarashi J, Greif D, Michel T. The regulation and pharmacology of endothelial nitric oxide synthase. Annu Rev Pharmacol Toxicol 46: 235–276, 2006. DOI: 10.1146/annurev.pharmtox.44.101802.121844 15

[102] Murad F. Shattuck Lecture. Nitric oxide and cyclic GMP in cell signaling and drug development. N Engl J Med 355: 2003–2011, 2006. DOI: 10.1056/NEJMsa063904 15

[103] Hess DT, Matsumoto A, Kim SO, Marshall HE, Stamler JS. Protein S-nitrosylation: purview and parameters. Nat Rev Mol Cell Biol 6: 150–166, 2005. DOI: 10.1038/nrm1569 15

[104] Radomski MW, Palmer RM, Moncada S. Endogenous nitric oxide inhibits human platelet adhesion to vascular endothelium. Lancet 2: 1057–1058, 1987. DOI: 10.1016/S0140-6736(87)91481-4 15

[105] Marcondes S, Cardoso MH, Morganti RP, Thomazzi SM, Lilla S, Murad F, De Nucci G, Antunes E. Cyclic GMP-independent mechanisms contribute to the inhibition of platelet adhesion by nitric oxide donor: a role for alpha-actinin nitration. Proc Natl Acad Sci USA 103: 3434–3439, 2006. DOI: 10.1073/pnas.0509397103 15

[106] Schafer A, Wiesmann F, Neubauer S, Eigenthaler M, Bauersachs J, Channon KM. Rapid regulation of platelet activation in vivo by nitric oxide. Circulation 109: 1819–1822, 2004. DOI: 10.1161/01.CIR.0000126837.88743.DD 15

[107] Cerwinka WH, Cooper D, Krieglstein CF, Feelisch M, Granger DN. Nitric oxide modulates endotoxin-induced platelet-endothelial cell adhesion in intestinal venules. Am J Physiol Heart Circ Physiol 282: H1111–H1117, 2002. 15, 16

[108] Morrell CN, Matsushita K, Chiles K, Scharpf RB, Yamakuchi M, Mason RJ, Bergmeier W, Mankowski JL, Baldwin WM, 3rd, Faraday N, Lowenstein CJ. Regulation of platelet granule exocytosis by S-nitrosylation. Proc Natl Acad Sci USA 102: 3782–3787, 2005. DOI: 10.1073/pnas.0408310102 15

[109] Broeders MA, Tangelder GJ, Slaaf DW, Reneman RS, oude Egbrink MG. Endogenous nitric oxide and prostaglandins synergistically counteract thromboembolism in arterioles but not in venules. Arterioscler Thromb Vasc Biol 21: 163–169, 2001. 16, 40

[110] Broeders MA, Tangelder GJ, Slaaf DW, Reneman RS, oude Egbrink MG. Endogenous nitric oxide protects against thromboembolism in venules but not in arterioles. Arterioscler Thromb Vasc Biol 18: 139–145, 1998. 16, 40

[111] Ozuyaman B, Godecke A, Kusters S, Kirchhoff E, Scharf RE, Schrader J. Endothelial nitric oxide synthase plays a minor role in inhibition of arterial thrombus formation. Thromb Haemost 93: 1161–1167, 2005. 16

[112] Wood KC, Hebbel RP, Lefer DJ, Granger DN. Critical role of endothelial cell-derived nitric oxide synthase in sickle cell disease-induced microvascular dysfunction. Free Radic Biol Med 40: 1443–1453, 2006. DOI: 10.1016/j.freeradbiomed.2005.12.015 16

[113] Kubes P, Suzuki M, Granger DN. Nitric oxide: an endogenous modulator of leukocyte adhesion. Proc Natl Acad Sci USA 88: 4651–4655, 1991. DOI: 10.1073/pnas.88.11.4651 16

[114] Sase K and Michel T. Expression of constitutive endothelial nitric oxide synthase in human blood platelets. Life Sci 57: 2049–2055, 1995. DOI: 10.1016/0024-3205(95)02191-K 16

[115] Naseem KM and Riba R. Unresolved roles of platelet nitric oxide synthase. J Thromb Haemost 6: 10–19, 2008. DOI: http://doi.wiley.com/10.1111/j.1538-7836.2007.02802.x 16

[116] Gambaryan S, Kobsar A, Hartmann S, Birschmann I, Kuhlencordt PJ, Muller-Esterl W, Lohmann SM, Walter U. NO-synthase-/NO-independent regulation of human and murine platelet soluble guanylyl cyclase activity. J Thromb Haemost 6: 1376–1384, 2008. DOI: 10.1111/j.1538-7836.2008.03014.x 16

[117] Gryglewski RJ. Prostacyclin among prostanoids. Pharmacol Rep 60: 3–11, 2008. 16, 23

[118] Mitchell JA, Ali F, Bailey L, Moreno L, Harrington LS. Role of nitric oxide and prostacy-clin as vasoactive hormones released by the endothelium. Exp Physiol 93: 141–147, 2008. DOI: 10.1113/expphysiol.2007.038588 16

[119] Higgs EA, Higgs GA, Moncada S, Vane JR. Prostacyclin (PGI2) inhibits the formation of platelet thrombi in arterioles and venules of the hamster cheek pouch. Br J Pharmacol 63: 535–539, 1978. 16

[120] Moncada S, Gryglewski R, Bunting S, Vane JR. An enzyme isolated from arteries transforms prostaglandin endoperoxides to an unstable substance that inhibits platelet aggregation. Nature 263: 663–665, 1976. DOI: 10.1038/263663a0 16

[121] Eriksson AC and Whiss PA. Measurement of adhesion of human platelets in plasma to protein surfaces in microplates. J Pharmacol Toxicol Methods 52: 356–365, 2005. DOI: 10.1016/j.vascn.2005.06.002 16

[122] Shanberge JN, Kajiwara Y, Quattrociocchi-Longe T. Effect of aspirin and iloprost on adhesion of platelets to intact endothelium in vivo. J Lab Clin Med 125: 96–101, 1995. 16

[123] Hantgan RR, Hindriks G, Taylor RG, Sixma JJ, de Groot PG. Glycoprotein Ib, von Wille-brand factor, and glycoprotein IIb:IIIa are all involved in platelet adhesion to fibrin in flowing whole blood. Blood 76: 345–353, 1990. 16

[124] Marcus AJ, Broekman MJ, Drosopoulos JH, Olson KE, Islam N, Pinsky DJ, Levi R. Role of CD39 (NTPDase-1) in thromboregulation, cerebroprotection, and cardioprotection. Semin Thromb Hemost 31: 234–246, 2005. DOI: 10.1055/s-2005-869528 16

[125] Fung CY, Marcus AJ, Broekman MJ, Mahaut-Smith MP. P2X(1) receptor inhibition and soluble CD39 administration as novel approaches to widen the cardiovascular therapeutic window. Trends Cardiovasc Med 19: 1–5, 2009. DOI: 10.1016/j.tcm.2009.01.005 16

[126] Reitsma S, Slaaf DW, Vink H, van Zandvoort MA, oude Egbrink MG. The endothelial glycocalyx: composition, functions, and visualization. Pflugers Arch 454: 345–359, 2007. DOI: 10.1007/s00424-007-0212-8 16

[127] Noble MI, Drake-Holland AJ, Vink H. Hypothesis: arterial glycocalyx dysfunction is the first step in the atherothrombotic process. Qjm 101: 513–518, 2008. DOI: 10.1093/qjmed/hcn024 17

[128] Vink H, Constantinescu AA, Spaan JA. Oxidized lipoproteins degrade the endothelial surface layer: implications for platelet-endothelial cell adhesion. Circulation 101: 1500–1502, 2000. 17

[129] van den Berg BM, Vink H, Spaan JA. The endothelial glycocalyx protects against myocardial edema. Circ Res 92: 592–594, 2003. DOI: 10.1161/01.RES.0000065917.53950.75 17

[130] Vink H and Duling BR. Identification of distinct luminal domains for macromolecules, erythrocytes, and leukocytes within mammalian capillaries. Circ Res 79: 581–589, 1996. 17

[131] Smith ML, Long DS, Damiano ER, Ley K. Near-wall micro-PIV reveals a hydrodynamically relevant endothelial surface layer in venules in vivo. Biophys J 85: 637–645, 2003. DOI: 10.1016/S0006-3495(03)74507-X 17

[132] Baldwin AL and Winlove CP. Effects of perfusate composition on binding of ruthenium red and gold colloid to glycocalyx of rabbit aortic endothelium. J Histochem Cytochem 32: 259–266, 1984. 17

[133] Weinbaum S, Tarbell JM, Damiano ER. The structure and function of the endothelial glycocalyx layer. Annu Rev Biomed Eng 9: 121–167, 2007. DOI: 10.1146/annurev.bioeng.9.060906.151959 17

[134] Rumbaut RE, Slaaf DW, Burns AR. Microvascular thrombosis models in venules and arterioles in vivo. Microcirculation 12: 259–274, 2005. DOI: 10.1080/10739680590925664 18, 25, 40

[135] Wood KC, Hebbel RP, Granger DN. Endothelial cell P-selectin mediates a proinflammatory and prothrombogenic phenotype in cerebral venules of sickle cell transgenic mice. Am J Physiol Heart Circ Physiol 286: H1608–1614, 2004. DOI: 10.1152/ajpheart.01056.2003 18

[136] Katayama T, Ikeda Y, Handa M, Tamatani T, Sakamoto S, Ito M, Ishimura Y, Suematsu M. Immunoneutralization of glycoprotein Ibalpha attenuates endotoxin-induced interactions of platelets and leukocytes with rat venular endothelium in vivo. Circ Res 86: 1031–1037, 2000. 18

[137] Cooper D, Russell J, Chitman KD, Williams MC, Wolf RE, Granger DN. Leukocyte dependence of platelet adhesion in postcapillary venules. Am J Physiol Heart Circ Physiol 286: H1895–1900, 2004. DOI: 10.1152/ajpheart.01000.2003 19

[138] Rumbaut RE, Bellera RV, Randhawa JK, Shrimpton CN, Dasgupta SK, Dong JF, Burns AR. Endotoxin enhances microvascular thrombosis in mouse cremaster venules via a TLR4-dependent, neutrophil-independent mechanism. Am J Physiol Heart Circ Physiol 290: H1671–1679, 2006. 19, 40

[139] Li Z, Rumbaut RE, Burns AR, Smith CW. Platelet response to corneal abrasion is necessary for acute inflammation and efficient re-epithelialization. Invest Ophthalmol Vis Sci 47: 4794–4802, 2006. DOI: 10.1167/iovs.06-0381 19

[140] Zarbock A, Polanowska-Grabowska RK, Ley K. Platelet-neutrophil-interactions: linking hemostasis and inflammation. Blood Rev 21: 99–111, 2007. 19

[141] Kuijper PH, Gallardo Tores HI, Lammers JW, Sixma JJ, Koenderman L, Zwaginga JJ. Platelet associated fibrinogen and ICAM-2 induce firm adhesion of neutrophils under flow conditions. Thromb Haemost 80: 443–448, 1998. 19

[142] Zarbock A, Singbartl K, Ley K. Complete reversal of acid-induced acute lung injury by blocking of platelet-neutrophil aggregation. J Clin Invest 116: 3211–3219, 2006. DOI: 10.1172/JCI29499 19

[143] Dong JF. Cleavage of ultra-large von Willebrand factor by ADAMTS-13 under flow conditions. J Thromb Haemost 3: 1710–1716, 2005. DOI: 10.1111/j.1538-7836.2005.01360.x 20

[144] Bernardo A, Ball C, Nolasco L, Moake JF, Dong JF. Effects of inflammatory cytokines on the release and cleavage of the endothelial cell-derived ultralarge von Willebrand factor multimers under flow. Blood 104: 100–106, 2004. 20

[145] Dong JF, Moake JL, Nolasco L, Bernardo A, Arceneaux W, Shrimpton CN, Schade AJ, McIntire LV, Fujikawa K, Lopez JA. ADAMTS-13 rapidly cleaves newly secreted ultralarge von Willebrand factor multimers on the endothelial surface under flowing conditions. Blood 100: 4033–4039, 2002. 20, 41

[146] Chauhan AK, Goerge T, Schneider SW, Wagner DD. Formation of platelet strings and microthrombi in the presence of ADAMTS-13 inhibitor does not require P-selectin or beta3 integrin. J Thromb Haemost 5: 583–589, 2007. DOI: 10.1111/j.1538-7836.2007.02361.x 20, 41

[147] Moake JL. Thrombotic microangiopathies. N Engl J Med 347: 589–600, 2002. DOI: 10.1056/NEJMra020528 20

[148] Nguyen TC, Liu A, Liu L, Ball C, Choi H, May WS, Aboulfatova K, Bergeron AL, Dong JF. Acquired ADAMTS-13 deficiency in pediatric patients with severe sepsis. Haematologica 92: 121–124, 2007. DOI: 10.3324/haematol.10262 20, 41

[149] Ono T, Mimuro J, Madoiwa S, Soejima K, Kashiwakura Y, Ishiwata A, Takano K, Ohmori T, Sakata Y. Severe secondary deficiency of von Willebrand factor-cleaving protease (ADAMTS13) in patients with sepsis-induced disseminated intravascular coagulation: its correlation with development of renal failure. Blood 107: 528–534, 2006. DOI: 10.1182/blood-2005-03-1087 20, 41

[150] Chauhan AK, Kisucka J, Brill A, Walsh MT, Scheiflinger F, Wagner DD. ADAMTS13: a new link between thrombosis and inflammation. J Exp Med 205: 2065–2074, 2008. DOI: 10.1084/jem.20080130 20

[151] da Costa Martins P, Garcia-Vallejo JJ, van Thienen JV, Fernandez-Borja M, van Gils JM, Beckers C, Horrevoets AJ, Hordijk PL, Zwaginga JJ. P-selectin glycoprotein ligand-1 is expressed on endothelial cells and mediates monocyte adhesion to activated endothelium. Arterioscler Thromb Vasc Biol 27: 1023–1029, 2007. DOI: 10.1161/ATVBAHA.107.140442 20

[152] Rivera-Nieves J, Burcin TL, Olson TS, Morris MA, McDuffie M, Cominelli F, Ley K. Critical role of endothelial P-selectin glycoprotein ligand 1 in chronic murine ileitis. J Exp Med 203: 907–917, 2006. DOI: 10.1084/jem.20052530 20

[153] Frenette PS, Denis CV, Weiss L, Jurk K, Subbarao S, Kehrel B, Hartwig JH, Vestweber D, Wagner DD. P-Selectin glycoprotein ligand 1 (PSGL-1) is expressed on platelets and can mediate platelet-endothelial interactions in vivo. J Exp Med 191: 1413–1422, 2000. DOI: 10.1084/jem.191.8.1413 20

[154] Massberg S, Enders G, Matos FC, Tomic LI, Leiderer R, Eisenmenger S, Messmer K, Krombach F. Fibrinogen deposition at the postischemic vessel wall promotes platelet adhesion during ischemia-reperfusion in vivo. Blood 94: 3829–3838, 1999. 20

[155] Khandoga A, Biberthaler P, Enders G, Axmann S, Hutter J, Messmer K, Krombach F. Platelet adhesion mediated by fibrinogen-intercellular adhesion molecule-1 binding induces tissue injury in the postischemic liver in vivo. Transplantation 74: 681–688, 2002. 20

[156] Varga-Szabo D, Braun A, Nieswandt B. Calcium signaling in platelets. J Thromb Haemost 7: 1057–1066, 2009. DOI: 10.1111/j.1538-7836.2009.03455.x 23

[157] Fox JE. Cytoskeletal proteins and platelet signaling. Thromb Haemost 86: 198–213, 2001. 23

[158] Escolar G, Krumwiede M, White JG. Organization of the actin cytoskeleton of resting and activated platelets in suspension. Am J Pathol 123: 86–94, 1986. 23

[159] Daniel JL, Molish IR, Rigmaiden M, Stewart G. Evidence for a role of myosin phosphorylation in the initiation of the platelet shape change response. J Biol Chem 259: 9826–9831, 1984. 23

[160] Jennings LK, Fox JE, Edwards HH, Phillips DR. Changes in the cytoskeletal structure of human platelets following thrombin activation. J Biol Chem 256: 6927–6932, 1981. 23

[161] Shattil SJ and Newman PJ. Integrins: dynamic scaffolds for adhesion and signaling in platelets. Blood 104: 1606–1615, 2004. DOI: 10.1182/blood-2004-04-1257 24

[162] Goto S, Ikeda Y, Saldivar E, Ruggeri ZM. Distinct mechanisms of platelet aggregation as a consequence of different shearing flow conditions. J Clin Invest 101: 479–486, 1998. DOI: 10.1172/JCI973 24

[163] Sobocka MB, Sobocki T, Babinska A, Hartwig JH, Li M, Ehrlich YH, Kornecki E. Signaling pathways of the F11 receptor (F11R; a.k.a. JAM-1, JAM-A) in human platelets: F11R dimerization, phosphorylation and complex formation with the integrin GPIIIa. J Recept Signal Transduct Res 24: 85–105, 2004. DOI: 10.1081/RRS-120034252 25

[164] Nanda N, Andre P, Bao M, Clauser K, Deguzman F, Howie D, Conley PB, Terhorst C, Phillips DR. Platelet aggregation induces platelet aggregate stability via SLAM family receptor signaling. Blood 106: 3028–3034, 2005. DOI: 10.1182/blood-2005-01-0333 25

[165] Andre P, Prasad KS, Denis CV, He M, Papalia JM, Hynes RO, Phillips DR, Wagner DD. CD40L stabilizes arterial thrombi by a beta3 integrin–dependent mechanism. Nat Med 8: 247–252, 2002. DOI: 10.1038/nm0302-247 25

[166] Rand ML, Leung R, Packham MA. Platelet function assays. Transfus Apher Sci 28: 307–317, 2003. DOI: 10.1016/S1473-0502(03)00050-8 25

[167] oude Egbrink MG, Tangelder GJ, Slaaf DW, Reneman RS. Thromboembolic reaction following wall puncture in arterioles and venules of the rabbit mesentery. Thromb Haemost 59: 23–28, 1988. 25, 40

[168] Falati S, Gross P, Merrill-Skoloff G, Furie BC, Furie B. Real-time in vivo imaging of platelets, tissue factor and fibrin during arterial thrombus formation in the mouse. Nature Med 8: 1175–1181, 2002. DOI: 10.1038/nm782 25

[169] Kuijpers MJ, Munnix IC, Cosemans JM, Vlijmen BV, Reutelingsperger CP, Egbrink MO, Heemskerk JW. Key role of platelet procoagulant activity in tissue factor-and collagen-dependent thrombus formation in arterioles and venules in vivo differential sensitivity to thrombin inhibition. Microcirculation 15: 269–282, 2008. DOI: 10.1080/10739680701653517 25

[170] Povlishock JT, Rosenblum WI, Sholley MM, Wei EP. An ultrastructural analysis of endothelial change paralleling platelet aggregation in a light/dye model of microvascular insult. Am J Pathol 110: 148–160, 1983. 26

[171] Ni H, Denis CV, Subbarao S, Degen JL, Sato TN, Hynes RO, Wagner DD. Persistence of platelet thrombus formation in arterioles of mice lacking both von Willebrand factor and fibrinogen. J Clin Invest 106: 385–392, 2000. DOI: 10.1172/JCI9896 26

[172] Vine AK. Recent advances in haemostasis and thrombosis. Retina 29: 1–7, 2009. 29

[173] Schenone M, Furie BC, Furie B. The blood coagulation cascade. Curr Opin Hematol 11: 272–277, 2004. DOI: 10.1097/01.moh.0000130308.37353.d4 29

[174] Ajjan R and Grant PJ. Coagulation and atherothrombotic disease. Atherosclerosis 186: 240–259, 2006. DOI: 10.1016/j.atherosclerosis.2005.10.042 29

[175] Kalafatis M, Swords NA, Rand MD, Mann KG. Membrane-dependent reactions in blood coagulation: role of the vitamin K-dependent enzyme complexes. Biochim Biophys Acta 1227: 113–129, 1994. 30

[176] Schroit AJ and Zwaal RF. Transbilayer movement of phospholipids in red cell and platelet membranes. Biochim Biophys Acta 1071: 313–329, 1991. 30

[177] Ahmad SS, Rawala-Sheikh R, Walsh PN. Components and assembly of the factor X activating complex. Semin Thromb Hemost 18: 311–323, 1992. DOI: 10.1055/s-2007-1002570 30

[178] Weiss HJ, Vicic WJ, Lages BA, Rogers J. Isolated deficiency of platelet procoagulant activity. Am J Med 67: 206–213, 1979. DOI: 10.1016/0002-9343(79)90392-9 31

[179] Rosing J, Bevers EM, Comfurius P, Hemker HC, van Dieijen G, Weiss HJ, Zwaal RF. Impaired factor X and prothrombin activation associated with decreased phospholipid exposure in platelets from a patient with a bleeding disorder. Blood 65: 1557–1561, 1985. 31

[180] Wolf P. The nature and significance of platelet products in human plasma. Br J Haematol 13: 269–288, 1967. DOI: 10.1111/j.1365-2141.1967.tb08741.x 31

[181] Crawford N. The presence of contractile proteins in platelet microparticles isolated from human and animal platelet-free plasma. Br J Haematol 21: 53–69, 1971. DOI: 10.1111/j.1365-2141.1971.tb03416.x 31

[182] Sims PJ, Wiedmer T, Esmon CT, Weiss HJ, Shattil SJ. Assembly of the platelet prothrombinase complex is linked to vesiculation of the platelet plasma membrane. Studies in Scott syndrome: an isolated defect in platelet procoagulant activity. J Biol Chem 264: 17049–17057, 1989. 31

[183] George JN, Pickett EB, Saucerman S, McEver RP, Kunicki TJ, Kieffer N, Newman PJ. Platelet surface glycoproteins. Studies on resting and activated platelets and platelet membrane microparticles in normal subjects, and observations in patients during adult respiratory distress syndrome and cardiac surgery. J Clin Invest 78: 340–348, 1986. DOI: 10.1172/JCI112582 31

[184] Warkentin TE and Sheppard JI. Generation of platelet-derived microparticles and proco-agulant activity by heparin-induced thrombocytopenia IgG/serum and other IgG platelet agonists: a comparison with standard platelet agonists. Platelets 10: 319–326, 1999. 31

[185] Galli M, Bevers EM, Comfurius P, Barbui T, Zwaal RF. Effect of antiphospholipid anti-bodies on procoagulant activity of activated platelets and platelet-derived microvesicles. Br J Haematol 83: 466–472, 1993. DOI: 10.1111/j.1365-2141.1993.tb04672.x 31

[186] Lee YJ, Jy W, Horstman LL, Janania J, Reyes Y, Kelley RE, Ahn YS. Elevated platelet microparticles in transient ischemic attacks, lacunar infarcts, and multiinfarct dementias. Thromb Res 72: 295–304, 1993. DOI: 10.1016/0049-3848(93)90138-E 31

[187] Kelton JG, Warkentin TE, Hayward CP, Murphy WG, Moore JC. Calpain activity in patients with thrombotic thrombocytopenic purpura is associated with platelet microparticles. Blood 80: 2246–2251, 1992. 31

[188] Baj-Krzyworzeka M, Majka M, Pratico D, Ratajczak J, Vilaire G, Kijowski J, Reca R, Janowska-Wieczorek A, Ratajczak MZ. Platelet-derived microparticles stimulate prolifer-ation, survival, adhesion, and chemotaxis of hematopoietic cells. Exp Hematol 30: 450–459, 2002. DOI: 10.1016/S0301-472X(02)00791-9 31

[189] Rozmyslowicz T, Majka M, Kijowski J, Murphy SL, Conover DO, Poncz M, Ratajczak J, Gaulton GN, Ratajczak MZ. Platelet- and megakaryocyte-derived microparticles transfer CXCR4 receptor to CXCR4-null cells and make them susceptible to infection by X4-HIV. Aids 17: 33–42, 2003. 31

[190] Merten M, Pakala R, Thiagarajan P, Benedict CR. Platelet microparticles promote platelet interaction with subendothelial matrix in a glycoprotein IIb/IIIa-dependent mechanism. Cir-culation 99: 2577–2582, 1999. 31

[191] Hrachovinova I, Cambien B, Hafezi-Moghadam A, Kappelmayer J, Camphausen RT, Widom A, Xia L, Kazazian HH, Jr., Schaub RG, McEver RP, Wagner DD. Interaction of P-selectin and PSGL-1 generates microparticles that correct hemostasis in a mouse model of hemophilia A. Nat Med 9: 1020–1025, 2003. DOI: 10.1038/nm899 31

[192] Mackman N. Role of tissue factor in hemostasis, thrombosis, and vas-cular development. Arterioscler Thromb Vasc Biol 24: 1015–1022, 2004. DOI: 10.1161/01.ATV.0000130465.23430.74 32

[193] Giesen PL, Rauch U, Bohrmann B, Kling D, Roque M, Fallon JT, Badimon JJ, Himber J, Riederer MA, Nemerson Y. Blood-borne tissue factor: another view of thrombosis. Proc Natl Acad Sci U S A 96: 2311–2315, 1999. DOI: 10.1073/pnas.96.5.2311 32

[194] Falati S, Liu Q, Gross P, Merrill-Skoloff G, Chou J, Vandendries E, Celi A, Croce K, Furie BC, Furie B. Accumulation of tissue factor into developing thrombi in vivo is dependent upon microparticle P-selectin glycoprotein ligand 1 and platelet P-selectin. J Exp Med 197: 1585–1598, 2003. DOI: 10.1084/jem.20021868 32

[195] Kumar A, Villani MP, Patel UK, Keith JC, Jr., Schaub RG. Recombinant soluble form of PSGL-1 accelerates thrombolysis and prevents reocclusion in a porcine model. Circulation 99: 1363–1369, 1999. 32

[196] Afshar-Kharghan V and Thiagarajan P. Leukocyte adhesion and thrombosis. Curr Opin Hematol 13: 34–39, 2006. DOI: 10.1097/01.moh.0000190107.54790.de 32, 34

[197] Del Conde I, Shrimpton CN, Thiagarajan P, Lopez JA. Tissue-factor-bearing microvesicles arise from lipid rafts and fuse with activated platelets to initiate coagulation. Blood 106: 1604–1611, 2005. 32

[198] Eilertsen KE and Osterud B. Tissue factor: (patho)physiology and cellular biology. Blood Coagul Fibrinolysis 15: 521–538, 2004. 32

[199] Satta N, Toti F, Feugeas O, Bohbot A, Dachary-Prigent J, Eschwege V, Hedman H, Freyssinet JM. Monocyte vesiculation is a possible mechanism for dissemination of membrane-associated procoagulant activities and adhesion molecules after stimulation by lipopolysaccharide. J Immunol 153: 3245–3255, 1994. 33

[200] Plescia J and Altieri DC. Activation of Mac-1 (CD11b/CD18)-bound factor X by released cathepsin G defines an alternative pathway of leucocyte initiation of coagulation. Biochem J 319 (Pt 3): 873–879, 1996. 34

[201] Si-Tahar M, Pidard D, Balloy V, Moniatte M, Kieffer N, Van Dorsselaer A, Chignard M. Human neutrophil elastase proteolytically activates the platelet integrin alphaIIbbeta3 through cleavage of the carboxyl terminus of the alphaIIb subunit heavy chain. Involvement in the potentiation of platelet aggregation. J Biol Chem 272: 11636–11647, 1997. 34

[202] May AE, Langer H, Seizer P, Bigalke B, Lindemann S, Gawaz M. Platelet-leukocyte interactions in inflammation and atherothrombosis. Semin Thromb Hemost 33: 123–127, 2007. DOI: 10.1055/s-2007-969023 34

[203] Lowe GD, Machado SG, Krol WF, Barton BA, Forbes CD. White blood cell count and haematocrit as predictors of coronary recurrence after myocardial infarction. Thromb Haemost 54: 700–703, 1985. 34

[204] Coller BS. Leukocytosis and ischemic vascular disease morbidity and mortality: is it time to intervene? Arterioscler Thromb Vasc Biol 25: 658–670, 2005. DOI: 10.1161/01.ATV.0000156877.94472.a5 34

[205] Heron M, Hoyert DL, Murphy SL, Xu J, Kochanek KD, Tejada-Vera B. Deaths: final data for 2006. Natl Vital Stat Rep 57: 1–134, 2009. 35

[206] Esmon CT. Basic mechanisms and pathogenesis of venous thrombosis. Blood Rev 23: 225–229, 2009. DOI: 10.1016/j.blre.2009.07.002 35

[207] Franchini M and Mannucci PM. Venous and arterial thrombosis: different sides of the same coin? Eur J Intern Med 19: 476–481, 2008. DOI: 10.1016/j.ejim.2007.10.019 35

[208] Lopez JA and Chen J. Pathophysiology of venous thrombosis. Thromb Res 123 Suppl 4: S30–34, 2009. DOI: 10.1016/S0049-3848(09)70140-9 35

[209] Aird WC. Vascular bed-specific thrombosis. J Thromb Haemost 5, Suppl 1: 283–291, 2007. DOI: http://doi.wiley.com/10.1111/j.1538-7836.2007.02515.x 35, 38

[210] Chan MY, Andreotti F, Becker RC. Hypercoagulable states in cardiovascular disease. Circulation 118: 2286–2297, 2008. DOI: 10.1161/CIRCULATIONAHA.108.778837 35, 37

[211] Heit JA. Venous thromboembolism: disease burden, outcomes and risk factors. J Thromb Haemost 3: 1611–1617, 2005. DOI: 10.1111/j.1538-7836.2005.01415.x 35

[212] Bagot CN and Arya R. Virchow and his triad: a question of attribution. Br J Haematol 143: 180–190, 2008. DOI: 10.1111/j.1365-2141.2008.07323.x 35

[213] Sevitt S. The structure and growth of valve-pocket thrombi in femoral veins. J Clin Pathol 27: 517–528, 1974. DOI: 10.1136/jcp.27.7.517 37

[214] Lopez JA, Kearon C, Lee AY. Deep venous thrombosis. Hematology Am Soc Hematol Educ Program: 439–456, 2004. 37

[215] Hamer JD, Malone PC, Silver IA. The PO2 in venous valve pockets: its possible bearing on thrombogenesis. Br J Surg 68: 166–170, 1981. DOI: 10.1002/bjs.1800680308 37

[216] Closse C, Seigneur M, Renard M, Pruvost A, Dumain P, Belloc F, Boisseau MR. Influence of hypoxia and hypoxia-reoxygenation on endothelial P-selectin expression. Thromb Res 85: 159–164, 1997. DOI: 10.1016/S0049-3848(96)00233-2 37

[217] Poredos P and Jezovnik MK. The role of inflammation in venous thromboembolism and the link between arterial and venous thrombosis. Int Angiol 26: 306–311, 2007. 37

[218] Di Nisio M, Wichers IM, Middeldorp S. Treatment for superficial thrombophlebitis of the leg. Cochrane Database Syst Rev: CD004982, 2007. 37

[219] Jacobs BR. Central venous catheter occlusion and thrombosis. Crit Care Clin 19: 489–514, ix, 2003. DOI: 10.1016/S0749-0704(03)00002-2 37

[220] Xiang DZ, Verbeken EK, Van Lommel AT, Stas M, De Wever I. Composition and formation of the sleeve enveloping a central venous catheter. J Vasc Surg 28: 260–271, 1998. DOI: 10.1016/S0741-5214(98)70162-4 37

[221] Raad, II, Luna M, Khalil SA, Costerton JW, Lam C, Bodey GP. The relationship between the thrombotic and infectious complications of central venous catheters. Jama 271: 1014–1016, 1994. DOI: 10.1001/jama.271.13.1014 37

[222] Lowe GDO, Greer IA, Cooke TG, Dewar EP, Evans MJ, Forbes CD, Mollan RAB, Scurr JH, de Swiet M. Risk of and prophylaxis for venous thromboembolism in hospital patients. Thromboembolic Risk Factors (THRIFT) Consensus Group. Bmj 305: 567–574, 1992. 38

[223] Culver D, Crawford JS, Gardiner JH, Wiley AM. Venous thrombosis after fractures of the upper end of the femur. A study of incidence and site. J Bone Joint Surg Br 52: 61–69, 1970. 38

[224] Scurr JH, Machin SJ, Bailey-King S, Mackie IJ, McDonald S, Smith PD. Frequency and prevention of symptomless deep-vein thrombosis in long-haul flights: a randomised trial. Lancet 357: 1485–1489, 2001. DOI: 10.1016/S0140-6736(00)04645-6 38

[225] Cooley BC, Szema L, Chen CY, Schwab JP, Schmeling G. A murine model of deep vein thrombosis: characterization and validation in transgenic mice. Thromb Haemost 94: 498–503, 2005. DOI: 10.1160/TH05-03-0170 38

[226] Myers D, Jr., Farris D, Hawley A, Wrobleski S, Chapman A, Stoolman L, Knibbs R, Strieter R, Wakefield T. Selectins influence thrombosis in a mouse model of experimental deep venous thrombosis. J Surg Res 108: 212–221, 2002. DOI: 10.1006/jsre.2002.6552 38

[227] Hayes MJ, Morris GK, Hampton JR. Lack of effect of bed rest and cigarette smoking on development of deep venous thrombosis after myocardial infarction. Br Heart J 38: 981–983, 1976. DOI: 10.1136/hrt.38.9.981 38

[228] Pinsky DJ, Naka Y, Liao H, Oz MC, Wagner DD, Mayadas TN, Johnson RC, Hynes RO, Heath M, Lawson CA, Stern DM. Hypoxia-induced exocytosis of endothelial cell Weibel-Palade bodies. A mechanism for rapid neutrophil recruitment after cardiac preservation. J Clin Invest 97: 493–500, 1996. DOI: 10.1172/JCI118440 38

[229] Yan SF, Pinsky DJ, Stern DM. A pathway leading to hypoxia-induced vascular fibrin deposition. Semin Thromb Hemost 26: 479–483, 2000. DOI: 10.1055/s-2000-13203 38

[230] Kessler CM. The link between cancer and venous thromboembolism: a review. Am J Clin Oncol 32: S3–7, 2009. DOI: 10.1097/COC.0b013e3181b01b17 38

[231] Geerts WH, Bergqvist D, Pineo GF, Heit JA, Samama CM, Lassen MR, Colwell CW. Prevention of venous thromboembolism: American College of Chest Physicians Evidence-Based Clinical Practice Guidelines (8th Edition). Chest 133: 381S–453S, 2008. DOI: 10.1378/chest.08-0656 38

[232] Blom JW, Doggen CJ, Osanto S, Rosendaal FR. Malignancies, prothrombotic mutations, and the risk of venous thrombosis. Jama 293: 715–722, 2005. DOI: 10.1001/jama.293.6.715 38

[233] Heit JA, O'Fallon WM, Petterson TM, Lohse CM, Silverstein MD, Mohr DN, Melton LJ, 3rd. Relative impact of risk factors for deep vein thrombosis and pulmonary embolism: a population-based study. Arch Intern Med 162: 1245–1248, 2002. DOI: 10.1001/archinte.162.11.1245 38

[234] Kasthuri RS, Taubman MB, Mackman N. Role of tissue factor in cancer. J Clin Oncol 27: 4834–4838, 2009. DOI: 10.1200/JCO.2009.22.6324 38

[235] Khorana AA, Ahrendt SA, Ryan CK, Francis CW, Hruban RH, Hu YC, Hostetter G, Harvey J, Taubman MB. Tissue factor expression, angiogenesis, and thrombosis in pancreatic cancer. Clin Cancer Res 13: 2870–2875, 2007. DOI: 10.1158/1078-0432.CCR-06-2351 38

[236] Caine GJ, Stonelake PS, Lip GY, Kehoe ST. The hypercoagulable state of malignancy: pathogenesis and current debate. Neoplasia 4: 465–473, 2002. DOI: 10.1038/sj.neo.7900263 38

[237] Kirkali Z and Van Poppel H. A critical analysis of surgery for kidney cancer with vena cava invasion. Eur Urol 52: 658–662, 2007. DOI: 10.1016/j.eururo.2007.05.009 38

[238] Thomas GM, Panicot-Dubois L, Lacroix R, Dignat-George F, Lombardo D, Dubois C. Cancer cell-derived microparticles bearing P-selectin glycoprotein ligand 1 accelerate thrombus formation in vivo. J Exp Med 206: 1913–1927, 2009. DOI: 10.1084/jem.20082297 38

[239] Ottinger H, Belka C, Kozole G, Engelhard M, Meusers P, Paar D, Metz KA, Leder LD, Cyrus C, Gnoth S, et al. Deep venous thrombosis and pulmonary artery embolism in high-grade non Hodgkin's lymphoma: incidence, causes and prognostic relevance. Eur J Haematol 54: 186–194, 1995. 38

[240] Bosson JL, Pouchain D, Bergmann JF. A prospective observational study of a cohort of outpatients with an acute medical event and reduced mobility: incidence of symptomatic thromboembolism and description of thromboprophylaxis practices. J Intern Med 260: 168–176, 2006. DOI: 10.1111/j.1365-2796.2006.01678.x 38

[241] Shivakumar SP, Anderson DR, Couban S. Catheter-associated thrombosis in patients with malignancy. J Clin Oncol 27: 4858–4864, 2009. DOI: 10.1200/JCO.2009.22.6126 38

[242] Shah PK. Inflammation and plaque vulnerability. Cardiovasc Drugs Ther 23: 31–40, 2009. DOI: 10.1007/s10557-008-6147-2 39

[243] Davies MJ, Richardson PD, Woolf N, Katz DR, Mann J. Risk of thrombosis in human atherosclerotic plaques: role of extracellular lipid, macrophage, and smooth muscle cell content. Br Heart J 69: 377–381, 1993. DOI: 10.1136/hrt.69.5.377 39

[244] Toschi V, Gallo R, Lettino M, Fallon JT, Gertz SD, Fernandez-Ortiz A, Chesebro JH, Badimon L, Nemerson Y, Fuster V, Badimon JJ. Tissue factor modulates the thrombogenicity of human atherosclerotic plaques. Circulation 95: 594–599, 1997. 39

[245] Badimon JJ, Lettino M, Toschi V, Fuster V, Berrozpe M, Chesebro JH, Badimon L. Local inhibition of tissue factor reduces the thrombogenicity of disrupted human atherosclerotic plaques: effects of tissue factor pathway inhibitor on plaque thrombogenicity under flow conditions. Circulation 99: 1780–1787, 1999. 39

[246] Essler M, Retzer M, Bauer M, Zangl KJ, Tigyi G, Siess W. Stimulation of platelets and endothelial cells by mildly oxidized LDL proceeds through activation of lysophosphatidic acid receptors and the Rho/Rho-kinase pathway. Inhibition by lovastatin. Ann N Y Acad Sci 905: 282–286, 2000. DOI: http://doi.wiley.com/10.1111/j.1749-6632.2000.tb06561.x 39

[247] Praprotnik S, Ferluga D, Vizjak A, Hvala A, Avcin T, Rozman B. Microthrombotic/microangiopathic manifestations of the antiphospholipid syndrome. Clin Rev Allergy Immunol 36: 109–125, 2009. DOI: 10.1007/s12016-008-8104-z 39

[248] Dalldorf FG and Jennette JC. Fatal Meningococcal septicemia. Arch Pahtol Lab Med 101: 6–9, 1977. 39

[249] Hosler GA, Cusumano AM, Hutchins GM. Thrombotic thrombocytopenic purpura and hemolytic uremic syndrome are distinct pathologic entities. A review of 56 autopsy cases. Arch Pathol Lab Med 127: 834–839, 2003. 39

[250] Hardaway RM. The significance of coagulative and thrombotic changes after haemorrhage and injury. J Clin Pathol Suppl (R Coll Pathol) 4: 110–120, 1970. DOI: 10.1136/jcp.s3-4.1.110 39

[251] oude Egbrink MG, van Gestel MA, Broeders MA, Tangelder GJ, Heemskerk JW, Reneman RS, Slaaf DW. Regulation of microvascular thromboembolism in vivo. Microcirculation 12, 2005. DOI: 10.1080/10739680590925628 40

[252] oude Egbrink MG, Tangelder GJ, Slaaf DW, Reneman RS. Different roles of prostaglandins in thromboembolic processes in arterioles and venules in vivo. Thromb Haemost 70: 826–833, 1993. 40

[253] Anthoni C, Russell J, Wood KC, Stokes KY, Vowinkel T, Kirchhofer D, Granger DN. Tissue factor: a mediator of inflammatory cell recruitment, tissue injury, and thrombus formation in experimental colitis. J Exp Med 204: 1595–1601, 2007. DOI: 10.1084/jem.20062354 40

[254] Sato M and Ohshima N. Effect of wall shear rate on thrombogenesis in microvessels of the rat mesentery. Circ Res 66: 941–949, 1990. 40

[255] oude Egbrink MG, Tangelder GJ, Slaaf DW, Reneman RS. Fluid dynamics and the thromboembolic reaction in mesenteric arterioles and venules. Am J Physiol 260: H1826–1833, 1991. 40

[256] Moake JL. von Willebrand factor, ADAMTS-13, and thrombotic thrombocytopenic purpura. Semin Hematol 41: 4–14, 2004. DOI: 10.1053/j.seminhematol.2003.10.003 41